苏州大学教材培育项目

医学基础形态学实验指导

（病理学分册）

主　审　李建明

主　编　邓　敏

苏州大学出版社

图书在版编目（CIP）数据

医学基础形态学实验指导．病理学分册／邓敏主编
．—苏州：苏州大学出版社，2019.12（2022.12重印）
苏州大学教材培育项目
ISBN 978-7-5672-3064-4

Ⅰ．①医… Ⅱ．①邓… Ⅲ．①人体形态学-实验-高
等学校-教学参考资料②病理学-实验-高等学校-教学
参考资料 Ⅳ．①R32-33②R36-33

中国版本图书馆 CIP 数据核字（2019）第 282326 号

Yixue Jichu Xingtaixue Shiyan Zhidao(Binglixue Fence)
书　　名：医学基础形态学实验指导（病理学分册）
主　　编：邓　敏
责任编辑：倪　青
出版发行：苏州大学出版社（Soochow University Press）
地　　址：苏州市十梓街 1 号　邮编：215006
印　　装：苏州市深广印刷有限公司
网　　址：http://www.sudapress.com
邮　　箱：sdcbs@suda.edu.cn
邮购热线：0512-67480030
销售热线：0512-67481020
开　　本：787mm×1 092mm　1/16　印张：12.25　字数：306 千
版　　次：2019 年 12 月第 1 版
印　　次：2022 年 12 月第 2 次印刷
书　　号：ISBN 978-7-5672-3064-4
定　　价：49.00 元

《医学基础形态学实验指导(病理学分册)》
编 委 会

主　　审　李建明

主　　编　邓　敏

副 主 编　刘　瑶

编　　委　(按姓氏笔画排序)

万　珊(苏州大学)

邓　敏(苏州大学)

刘　瑶(苏州大学)

郭玲玲(苏州大学)

董　亮(苏州大学)

谢　芳(苏州大学)

前　言

　　病理学是基础医学与临床医学之间非常重要的桥梁学科,是医学基础形态学的重要组成部分,是理论性和实践性都很强的课程。

　　病理学实验课程是病理学教学中非常重要的组成部分。在"互联网＋"时代,实验教学的形式和内容的改变是必然的。为了顺应时代的发展要求,苏州大学病理学与病理生理学系的老师发挥集体智慧,合力编写了这本《医学基础形态学实验指导(病理学分册)》。本教材在理论与实验相结合、基础与临床相结合、实体实验与虚拟实验相结合的总体原则指导下,主要从形态学角度引导学生主动学习,以提高学生自主学习的能力。

　　《医学基础形态学实验指导(病理学分册)》是基于苏州大学病理学与病理生理学系自有的实验标本编写完成的。它具有以下特点:

　　1. 实用性强。实验大体标本、组织切片均为苏州大学病理学与病理生理学系多年积累的典型实体标本,均为常见病、多发病,具有很强的实用性。

　　2. 图文并茂。书中插入了大量的相应病变的大体标本及组织切片图,对主要的病变图中均有标注。

　　3. 双语化。中英文双语对应,既利于提高中国学生的英文水平,又适用于医学留学生的教学。

　　4. 数字化。图书最后配有部分章节大体标本二维码,学生可以通过扫描二维码进行在线观察与学习。

　　5. 虚实结合。图书在介绍实体实验的基础上,增设了苏州大学虚拟实验的网址(http://mvl.suda.edu.cn/virlab/),学生可以在线学习相关的虚拟实验。

　　6. 理论与实验相结合。在实验指导中,结合相应的病理改变,提出了相关的理论问题。

　　7. 基础与临床相结合。每章都有病例分析,旨在提高学生分析问题与解决问题的能力,同时加深学生对理论知识的理解和应用。

　　本实验教材的内容基本与由步宏、李一雷主编的全国高等学校医学规划教材《病理学》相对应,并参考了苏州大学教授冯一中主编的《医学形态学实验指导》中病理学部分的内容。在此谨向冯一中教授及该书的编写人员表示感谢! 在本书的编写工作中,我们得到了本系各位老师、苏州大学医学部实验中心的顾永平老师以及部分本科学生的帮助和支持,在此对他们一并表示衷心的感谢!

　　由于我们的专业水平有限,书中如有错误或不妥之处,恳请各位同行专家和读者提出宝贵意见与建议,以便再版时订正。

本书编委会

2019 年 9 月

目 录

■ **绪论**

Introduction

    一、实验课的目的 The purpose of experimental course　／1

    二、实验内容及方法 The content and method of experiments　／1

    三、实验报告 The experimental report　／7

■ **第一章　细胞和组织适应与损伤**

Chapter 1　Cell and Tissue Adaptation and Injury

    一、教学目的 Teaching objectives　／10

    二、大体标本观察 Observation of gross specimens　／10

    三、组织切片观察 Observation of tissue slides　／16

    四、病例讨论 Case discussion　／23

    五、思考题 Questions　／23

■ **第二章　损伤的修复**

Chapter 2　Tissue Repair

    一、教学目的 Teaching objectives　／25

    二、大体标本观察 Observation of gross specimens　／25

    三、组织切片观察 Observation of tissue slides　／27

    四、病例讨论 Case discussion　／28

    五、思考题 Questions　／28

■ **第三章　局部血液循环障碍**

Chapter 3　Local Hemodynamic Disorder

    一、教学目的 Teaching objectives　／30

    二、大体标本观察 Observation of gross specimens　／30

    三、组织切片观察 Observation of tissue slides　／37

    四、动物实验：家兔脂肪栓塞 Animal experiment：fat embolism in rabbits　／41

    五、病例讨论 Case discussion　／42

    六、思考题 Questions　／43

■ 第四章　炎症

Chapter 4　Inflammation

一、教学目的 Teaching objectives　/ 44

二、大体标本观察 Observation of gross specimens　/ 44

三、组织切片观察 Observation of tissue slides　/ 51

四、病例讨论 Case discussion　/ 53

五、思考题 Questions　/ 54

■ 第五章　肿瘤

Chapter 5　Tumors

一、教学目的 Teaching objectives　/ 55

二、大体标本观察 Observation of gross specimens　/ 55

三、组织切片观察 Observation of tissue slides　/ 72

四、病例讨论 Case discussion　/ 78

五、思考题 Questions　/ 79

■ 第六章　心血管系统疾病

Chapter 6　Diseases of the Heart and Blood Vessels System

一、教学目的 Teaching objectives　/ 81

二、大体标本观察 Observation of gross specimens　/ 81

三、组织切片观察 Observation of tissue slides　/ 87

四、病例讨论 Case discussion　/ 91

五、思考题 Questions　/ 92

■ 第七章　呼吸系统疾病

Chapter 7　Diseases of the Respiratory System

一、教学目的 Teaching objectives　/ 93

二、大体标本观察 Observation of gross specimens　/ 93

三、组织切片观察 Observation of tissue slides　/ 99

四、病例讨论 Case discussion　/ 103

五、思考题 Questions　/ 104

■ 第八章 消化系统疾病
Chapter 8 Diseases of the Digestive System

一、教学目的 Teaching objectives / 106

二、大体标本观察 Observation of gross specimens / 106

三、组织切片观察 Observation of tissue slides / 117

四、病例讨论 Case discussion / 122

五、思考题 Questions / 124

■ 第九章 淋巴造血系统疾病
Chapter 9 Disorders of the Hematopoietic and Lymphoid System

一、教学目的 Teaching objectives / 126

二、大体标本观察 Observation of gross specimens / 126

三、组织切片观察 Observation of tissue slides / 127

四、病例讨论 Case discussion / 128

五、思考题 Questions / 129

■ 第十章 泌尿系统疾病
Chapter 10 Diseases of the Urinary System

一、教学目的 Teaching objectives / 130

二、大体标本观察 Observation of gross specimens / 130

三、组织切片观察 Observation of tissue slides / 133

四、病例讨论 Case discussion / 136

五、思考题 Questions / 137

■ 第十一章 生殖系统疾病与乳腺疾病
Chapter 11 Diseases of the Genital System and the Breast

一、教学目的 Teaching objectives / 138

二、大体标本观察 Observation of gross specimens / 138

三、组织切片观察 Observation of tissue slides / 143

四、病例讨论 Case discussion / 145

五、思考题 Questions / 146

■ 第十二章　内分泌系统(甲状腺)疾病

Chapter 12　Diseases of the Endocrine System（Thyroid）

一、教学目的 Teaching objectives　／147

二、大体标本观察 Observation of gross specimens　／147

三、组织切片观察 Observation of tissue slides　／149

四、病例讨论 Case discussion　／150

五、思考题 Questions　／151

■ 第十三章　神经系统疾病

Chapter 13　Diseases of the Nervous System

一、教学目的 Teaching objectives　／152

二、大体标本观察 Observation of gross specimens　／152

三、组织切片观察 Observation of tissue slides　／152

四、思考题 Questions　／154

■ 第十四章　感染性疾病

Chapter 14　Infectious Diseases

一、教学目的 Teaching objectives　／155

二、大体标本观察 Observation of gross specimens　／155

三、组织切片观察 Observation of tissue slides　／167

四、病例讨论 Case discussion　／171

五、思考题 Questions　／172

■ **附录　部分章节大体标本二维码**　／174

■ **参考文献**　／187

绪　论
Introduction

一、 实验课的目的 The purpose of experimental course

病理学是医学科学中重要的基础学科之一,是医学基础与临床之间的桥梁学科。病理学实验课是病理学教学中非常重要的组成部分,它主要是从形态学的角度,用直观的方法观察病变,对病变做出诊断,并进一步研究疾病的发生和发展规律。学生通过实验课对病变的大体标本和组织切片的观察,能更好地理解和掌握理论课所学过的基本理论知识,这样理论联系实践,培养学生分析问题和解决实际问题的能力。同时,实验方法的介绍和学习有助于培养学生的基本科研技能和科学态度。

Pathology is one of the important disciplines in basic medicine, as well as a bridge between basic and clinical medicine. The pathology experiment class is a crucial part during teaching. It mainly observes the lesions from the perspective of morphology, diagnoses the lesions, and further studies the occurrence and development of the disease. Students can better understand and master the key part of the theoretical course by observing the diseased gross specimens and corresponding tissue slides in the experimental course, so that the theory can be linked to practice and the students' ability to analyze and solve practical problems could be promoted. At the same time, the introduction and learning of experimental methods can cultivate students' basic scientific research skills, ability and scientific attitude.

二、 实验内容及方法 The content and method of experiments

病理学实验课的内容主要包括大体标本的观察和诊断、组织切片的观察和诊断、动物实验、临床病理讨论、虚拟仿真实验及实验慕课学习五个方面。

The content of the experimental pathology course includes mainly the following aspects：Observation and diagnosis of gross specimens, observation and diagnosis of tissue slides, animal experiments, clinicopathological discussion, virtual simulation experiment and experimental MOOC learning.

（一）大体标本的观察和诊断 Observation and diagnosis of gross specimens

1. 标本的固定 Fixation of specimens

所有大体标本均来源于手术切除或尸体解剖,用10%的中性福尔马林(4%的甲醛水溶液)进行固定,并密封于标本盒内。固定液无色透明,但具有强烈的刺激性,因此在观察标本时请注意保持标本盒的密闭性。标本和组织固定后能保持其结构的完整性,但失去了其新鲜标本的颜色。大体标本常呈灰白色,血液常呈暗黑褐色。

All gross specimens were obtained from surgical resection or autopsy, fixed with 10% neutral formalin (4% formaldehyde) and sealed in the specimen box. The fixative solution is colorless and transparent, but highly irritative, therefore, please pay attention to keep the specimen box tight when observing specimens. Specimens and tissues can maintain their structural integrity after being fixed, but lose the original color of their fresh specimens. Gross specimens are often grayish-white and the blood is often dark brown after being fixed.

2. 观察方法和要点 Observation methods and main points

首先确认标本是何脏器或组织,然后从外向内、从上到下观察器官的体积、形状、颜色、硬度、表面及切面等是否有所改变,运用所学的理论知识找出病变的部位,进行综合分析并做出病理诊断。病理诊断的命名包括器官或组织名称加上病变或疾病名称:在总论部分常用病变名称,如肝脂肪变性;在各论部分则用疾病名称,如病毒性肝炎。

Firstly, confirm the specimen or tissue, and then observe its volume, shape, color, hardness, surface and section of the organ from the outside to the inside, from top to bottom, and use the theoretical knowledge to find the lesion, and conduct a comprehensive analysis to make the pathological diagnosis. The nomenclature of pathological diagnosis includes the name of the organ or tissue and the name of the pathological change or the diseases. In the general pathology, the pathological change like hepatic steatosis, is often used. While in the systemic pathology, the name of the disease is used, such as viral hepatitis.

（1）体积:有无增大或缩小。观察完整标本,增大时包膜紧张,缩小时则包膜皱缩;观察标本切面时,如器官增大,邻近包膜处可见边缘外翻。空腔器官需要注意其管壁的厚薄、管腔是否扩大或缩小。

Volume：Whether there is enlargement or reduction. Observe the whole specimen, the capsule is tight when enlarging, and shrinks when it is reduced. When the specimen is cut, the edge of the capsule turns outward near the capsule if the organ is enlarged. If it is a hollow organ, please pay attention to the thickness of its wall and whether the lumen is enlarged or reduced.

（2）形状：有无异常，有无新生物，其形态如何。

Shape：Whether there is an abnormality, whether there is any neoplasm, and its morphology.

（3）颜色、光泽：因标本已被固定，它原来的色泽受到影响。标本呈灰黄或灰白色。正常结构消失常为坏死的表现。组织暗红色常为淤血或出血；黄色常表示含有脂质成分；黑色则表示可能含有黑色素；黄绿色则表示可能含有胆汁成分。

Color and gloss：The original color is affected because the specimen has been fixed. The specimen is gray-yellow or gray-white. The normal structure disappears often as a manifestation of necrosis. Dark red tissue is often congested or hemorrhagic. Yellow tissue often indicates lipid content. Black tissue may contain melanin. Yellow-green tissue may contain bile components.

（4）表面：是否光滑，被膜有无渗出物或增厚；血管有无扩张、充血；被膜是否易于剥离。如果我们观察大脑组织表面，则应注意其脑回与脑沟是否清晰等。

Surface：Whether it is smooth. Whether there is exudates or thickening of the capsule. Whether the blood vessels are dilated or congested. Whether the capsule is easy to peel off. If we observe the surface of the brain tissue, we should notice whether the gyrus and sulcus are clear.

（5）切面：结构、颜色和质地有无改变，空腔脏器有无内容物，腔有无扩张或变小。

Cut surface：Whether there are any changes in structure, color and texture. Whether there are contents in the hollow organ. Whether the cavity expands or becomes small.

（6）病灶的情况：发现局限性病灶时，注意观察病灶的部位、分布、数目、形状、大小、颜色、质地、有无包膜及其与周围组织的关系等。

The lesion：When the localized lesion is found, pay attention to its location, distribution, number, shape, size, color, texture, presence or absence of the capsule and its relationship with the surrounding tissue.

（二）组织切片的观察和诊断 Observation and diagnosis of tissue slides

1. 组织切片的制作 Production of tissue slides

（1）苏木素-伊红（HE）染色：我们观察的组织切片大部分为此种染色。组织经取材、固定、脱水、石蜡包埋、切片、染色等过程，最终细胞核被染成蓝色，胞质呈淡红色。

Hematoxylin-eosin（HE）staining：Most of the tissue slides we observed are stained by this technique. The tissues are harvested, fixed, dehydrated, embedded in paraffin, sectioned, stained, etc. Finally, the nuclei are stained blue and the cytoplasm light red.

（2）特殊染色：在某些情况下，一般的 HE 染色无法满足病变观察的要求，我们可以采用其他的染色方法来显示病变,如苏丹染液染色可以显示脂质成分,过碘酸希夫(PAS)染色可以显示糖蛋白,银染可以显示网状纤维,普鲁士蓝染色可以显示铁离子,免疫组织化学染色可以显示各种抗原等。

Special staining：In some cases, general hematoxylin-eosin (HE) staining cannot meet the need of the observation of lesions, so we can use other staining methods to display lesions, such as Sudan staining to show lipid composition, periodic acid-Schiff (PAS) staining to show glycoprotein, silver staining to show reticular fibers, Prussian blue staining to show iron ions, and immunohistochemical staining can show various antigens.

2. 观察方法和要点 Observation methods and main points

(1)肉眼观察:首先在肉眼下初步观察,主要观察组织的大小、块数,染色是否均匀,密度等是否一致,以了解切片中病变部位及其大致情况。然后再用显微镜,按先低倍后高倍的顺序观察。

Visual inspection：First, make a preliminary observation with naked eyes. The main observation is the size and number of blocks, dyeing uniformity, density and so on, in order to understand the pathological changes in the slide and its general conditions. Then use a microscope to observe in the order of low magnification and high magnification.

(2)低倍镜观察:首先将切片的正面(有盖玻片的一面)放在4倍物镜下,从组织的边缘开始从左到右,自上而下,然后换一个视野再自下而上观察整个组织切片(图1),获得一个较为全面的印象,如什么组织或器官,与正常组织有何不同,从而找出病变部位,确定病变范围以及病变与周围组织之间的关系。

Low magnification observation：First, put the front side of the slide (with one side of the coverslip) under the 4 × objective, starting from the edge of the tissue, left to right, top to bottom, and then change the field of vision to observe the whole tissue slide from bottom to top (Fig. 1), and get a more comprehensive impression, such as what tissue or organ, the difference between the normal tissues and the lesion, and determine the extent of the lesion and its relationship with the surrounding tissue.

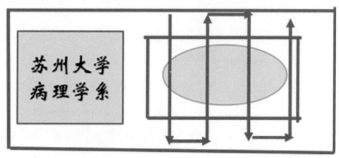

图 1　组织切片的观察顺序

Fig. 1　Observation order of tissue slides

（3）高倍镜观察：在低倍镜下找到并观察病变部位后，再用高倍物镜做进一步观察。此时主要观察组织和细胞病变的微细结构和形态，以进一步明确病变的性质。

High magnification observation：After the lesion is found，it is further observed with a high-power objective. At this time，the microstructure and morphology of the tissue and cytopathic lesions are mainly observed to further clarify the nature of the lesion.

（4）反复进行高低倍镜的交替观察，直至最后确认病变。

Repeat the observation of the high and low magnification lens until the lesion is finally confirmed.

※ 观察大体标本和组织切片的注意事项 Notices for observing gross specimens and tissue slides

（1）理论与实验的联系：在标本的观察中，需要将理论知识与实际的标本结合起来观察，通过实验，进一步巩固对理论知识的理解。

Combine theory with experiment：In the observation of specimens，it is necessary to combine theoretical knowledge with actual specimens，and further consolidate the understanding of theoretical knowledge through experiments.

（2）大体与镜下的联系：观察大体标本的病变需要考虑到显微镜下可能发生了哪些改变；反之，观察显微镜下组织学病变时，需要思考大体标本可能会出现哪些改变。如此，从宏观到微观或从微观到宏观更扎实地掌握各种知识。

Combine the gross with microscopic changes：When observing the pathological changes of gross specimens，we need to consider what changes may occur under the microscope；conversely，when observing histological changes under the microscope，it is necessary to consider what changes may occur in the gross specimens，so that we can master the knowledge more firmly from macro to micro or from micro to macro.

（3）形态与机能、基础与临床的联系：病理学主要通过形态学改变来研究疾病，但是我们一定要注意形态变化必然与功能及代谢的变化密切相关，从而推导出病人可能出现哪些功能障碍，出现哪些临床表现，将病理学基础知识与临床密切联系，这样可以提高病理学理论知识水平及其应用能力。

Combine morphology with function，basic and clinic medicine：Pathology mainly studies diseases from the aspect of morphological changes，but we must pay attention to the fact that morphological changes are closely related to changes in function and metabolism，so as to deduce which functional disorders may occur and which clinical manifestations may occur in patients，and to keep the basic knowledge of pathology closely related to clinic. Closely linking the basic knowledge of pathology with clinical practice can improve the theoretical knowledge and application ability of pathology.

（4）动态病变与静止标本的联系：人体的病变是一个动态发展的过程，而我们所观察到的切片或大体标本仅仅是其中静止的一部分，所以要学会综合分析，动静结合，进一步理解病变的发生发展规律。

Combine dynamic lesions with stationary specimens：The lesions of human body is a dynamic process，and the slides or macroscopic specimens we observe are only a static part，so we should learn to analyze comprehensively，combine the dynamics with the statics，with the further understand the occurrence and development of lesions.

（5）观察标本和切片时要细致、客观、全面。同一标本或切片中观察到两种或两种以上病变时，要分析它们的性质及其相互关系；不要丢大放小或丢小放大，要在理论知识的指导下实事求是地描述病变的特点，然后进行科学的分析和推理，做出正确的诊断。

When observing specimens and slides，it is necessary to be meticulous，objective and comprehensive. If two or more kinds of pathological changes are observed in the same specimen or slide，we need to analyze their nature and their relationship. We should not ignore large or small part of lesions，we need to describe the characteristics of pathological changes realistically and scientifically under the guidance of theoretical knowledge，and make a correct diagnosis through scientific analysis and reasoning.

（6）观察切片时，切忌一开始就盲目使用高倍物镜，这样容易损坏镜片和切片，又不能全面观察和分析切片中的病变，甚至遗漏重要病变，造成诊断上的错误；此外，一般病理切片观察不采用油镜。

When observing slides，do not blindly use high-power objective lens at the beginning，which is easy to damage the lens and the slides，and cannot fully observe，and analyze the lesions in the slides，or even miss important lesions，resulting in errors in diagnosis；in addition，general pathological slide observation does not use oil lens.

（7）标本和切片制作过程中可能出现多种人为现象，如切片中刀痕、福尔马林色素等，观察时要善于分辨，去伪存真，取其精华，抓住要点。

There may be many artificial phenomena in the process of making specimens and slides，such as knife marks in the slides，formalin pigment and so on. When observing，you need to be good at distinguishing，eliminating the false and taking the essence，and to master the main points.

（8）病理学实验课课前要预习相关的病理学理论知识，同时要复习解剖学、组织学、病原生物学及免疫学等知识。

Before the pathology experiment lesson，you need to preview the relevant pathology theory，at the same time，you need to review related knowledge about anatomy，histology，pathogenic biology，immunology and so on.

（三）动物实验 Animal experiments

病理学研究方法有很多。动物实验是不可或缺的重要部分,同时也是培养学生科研基本技能和动手能力的重要方法。在病理学实验课中会安排 1 ~ 2 次动物实验,让学生通过动态的观察进一步理解病变的发生发展规律。

There are many research methods in pathology. The experiment on animals is indispensable. It is also an important method to cultivate students' basic scientific research skills and practical ability. There will be 1 − 2 experiments on animals in pathology experiment, so that students can further understand the occurrence and development of some pathological changes through dynamic observation.

（四）临床病理讨论 Clinicopathological discussion

每章有 1 ~ 2 个临床病例讨论,通过分析典型病例的临床资料、实验室检查或者尸检资料,运用所学的病理学知识,在教师指导下进行讨论,理论联系实际,加深对所学知识的理解,以培养综合分析问题和解决问题的能力。

There are 1 − 2 clinical case discussions in each chapter. By analyzing the clinical data, laboratory examination or autopsy data of typical cases, using the pathological knowledge learned and under the guidance of teachers, you can combine theory with practice and deepen your understanding of the knowledge learned, and develop the ability to analyze and solve problems.

（五）虚拟仿真实验及实验慕课学习 Virtual simulation experiment and experimental MOOC learning

在“互联网 + ”时代,病理学实验教学中利用“互联网 + ”的优势将极大提高实验的教学效果。我们制作了几项虚拟仿真实验,拍摄了病理学实验慕课,作为病理学实验的辅助学习内容。学生通过自学这些知识,可以更好地学好病理学,为以后的临床学习打下良好的理论基础。

In the era of Internet plus, the advantage of Internet plus in pathological experiments will improve the teaching effects of experiments. We have made several virtual simulation experiments and photographed the pathology experiment as a supplementary study of pathological experiments. Students can learn pathology better by self-learning the knowledge, and lay a good theoretical foundation for future clinical learning.

三、 实验报告 The experimental report

书写实验报告的目的在于培养学生观察病变、认识病变、分析问题的能力和文字表达能力。它也是教师了解学生对病理知识的掌握情况，及时发现和解决教学中存在问题的重要途径之一。

The purpose of writing experiment reports is to cultivate students' ability of observing pathological changes, recognizing pathological lesions, analyzing problems and writing skills. It is also one of the important ways for teachers to understand students' mastery of pathological knowledge, and to find and solve problems during teaching in time.

实验报告的形式包括对大体标本、组织切片中的病变特点的描述，以及临床病例讨论的分析，以进一步加深对理论知识的理解。

The form of experiment reports includes the description of the pathological features of the gross specimen and tissue slides, and the analysis of the discussion of clinical cases to further deepen the understanding of theoretical knowledge.

组织切片图要求图片清晰、病变典型，并加以文字注释；描述病变应全面准确、突出重点、文字简练、条理清楚。

Tissue slide photography requires clear pictures, typical lesions, and text annotations. Describing lesions should be comprehensive and accurate, and key points need to be highlighted, concise and clearly described.

具体的病理学实验报告模板见图2。

Detailed pathology experiment report template is shown in Fig. 2.

苏州大学医学部病理学实验报告
Pathology Experiment Report of Medical College of Soochow University

姓名：　　　　　　　　专业：　　　　　　　　学号：
Name：　　　　　　　　Profession：　　　　　　Student number：

实验内容 Experiment content：

切片观察或大体标本描写 Slide observation or general specimen description：

图 1（插入图片）　Fig. 1（insert image）

图 2（插入图片）　Fig. 2（insert image）

诊断及诊断依据 Diagnosis and diagnostic basis：

得分 Score：

指导教师 Instructor：

日期 Date：

图 2　病理学实验报告模板
Fig. 2　Pathology experiment report template

编写 Written by：邓敏 Deng Min

英文审校 English proofreader：刘瑶 Liu Yao

第一章 细胞和组织适应与损伤

Chapter 1　Cell and Tissue Adaptation and Injury

一、 教学目的 Teaching objectives

（1）掌握适应性改变的概念，熟悉形态学特征及其对机体的影响。

Master the concept of adaptive changes, and be familiar with morphological features and their impacts on the body.

（2）掌握几种常见可逆性损伤（变性）的形态特点。

Master the morphologic changes of several common reversible injuries（degeneration）.

（3）掌握坏死的基本病变以及各种坏死类型的形态特点。

Master the basic lesions of necrosis, and various types of morphologic characters.

（4）熟悉坏死的结局。

Be familiar with the outcome of necrosis.

二、 大体标本观察 Observation of gross specimens

（一）适应 Adaptation

1. 萎缩 Atrophy

（1）肾萎缩（肾盂积水，图1-01）：肾脏体积增大，肾盂及肾盏极度扩张（★），肾实质显著变薄（➡）。

思考：该肾脏体积增大，为何仍称萎缩？属于哪种类型的萎缩？

Renal atrophy（renal hydronephrosis, Fig. 1-01）: The kidney is enlarged, the renal pelvis and renal calices are extremely dilated（★）, and the renal parenchyma is significantly thinner（➡）.

Question: Why the kidney is still called atrophy in spite of the enlargement of its size? What type of atrophy does it belong to?

（2）脑积水（图 1-02）：两侧脑室极度扩张如囊状（★），脑实质极度萎缩变薄（➡）。

思考：导致脑积水的原因有哪些？

Hydrocephalus (Fig. 1-02): The bilateral ventricles are extremely dilated, such as a cyst (★), and the brain parenchyma is extremely atrophied and thinned(➡).

Question:What are the causes of hydrocephalus?

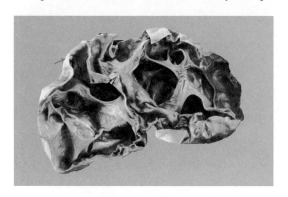
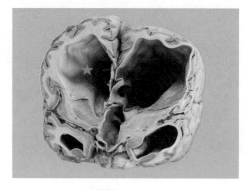

图 1-01 肾盂积水   图 1-02 脑积水

Fig. 1-01   Renal hydronephrosis   Fig. 1-02   Hydrocephalus

（3）心脏褐色萎缩（图 1-03）：成人心脏，体积明显缩小，颜色呈棕褐色，表面的冠状动脉由于心脏萎缩而蜿蜒迂曲（➡），心尖较锐（★）。

Heart brown atrophy (Fig. 1-03): Adult heart, the volume is significantly reduced, the color is brown. On the surface the coronary arteries are tortuous (➡) due to atrophy of the heart, and the apex is sharp(★).

2. 肥大 Hypertrophy

左心室肥大（图 1-04）：心脏体积明显增大，左心室壁肥厚（★）（正常厚 0.8～1.2 cm），乳头肌（➡）和肉柱均明显增厚，心尖圆钝。

思考：导致左心室肥大的常见原因有哪些？

Left ventricular hypertrophy (Fig. 1-04): The heart volume increased significantly, the left ventricular wall is hypertrophy (★) (normal thickness 0.8 – 1.2 cm), the papillary muscle (➡) and meat column were significantly thickened, and its apex is blunt.

Question:What are the common causes of left ventricular hypertrophy?

3. 增生 Hyperplasia

前列腺增生症（图 1-05）：前列腺体积增大，重量增加，切面可见灰白色实性结节（★），伴小囊（➡）形成。

Benign prostatic hyperplasia (Fig. 1-05): The prostate is enlarged in volume, the weight is increased, and the section of the prostate are visible with grayish solid nodules(★), with small sac formation（➡）.

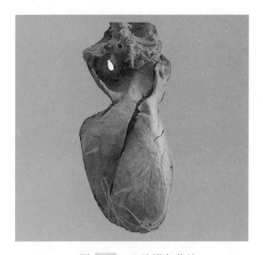

图 1-03　心脏褐色萎缩

Fig. 1-03　Heart brown atrophy

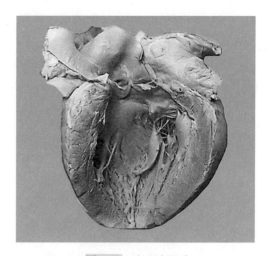

图 1-04　左心室肥大

Fig. 1-04　Left ventricular hypertrophy

（二）可逆性损伤——变性 Reversible injury—degeneration

1. 细胞水肿（水变性）Cellular swelling（Hydropic degeneration）

（1）肾脏细胞水肿（图 1-06）：儿童肾脏体积增大，边缘圆钝，包膜紧张，颜色苍白，切面肾皮质增宽（★），邻近包膜处外翻。

Renal cellular edema（Fig. 1-06）：The kid's kidney is enlarged with obtunded edges, tense capsule and pale in color. On the section, the cortex of the kidney is widened（★）and everted outward the capsule.

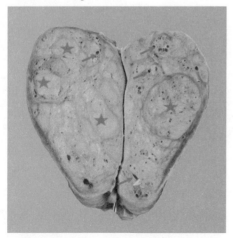

图 1-05　前列腺增生症

Fig. 1-05　Benign prostatic hyperplasia

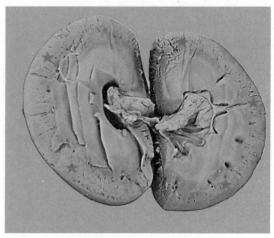

图 1-06　肾脏细胞水肿

Fig. 1-06　Renal cellular edema

（2）肝细胞水肿（图 1-07）：肝脏体积增大，包膜紧张，切面灰白、浑浊、无光泽。

Hepatocyte edema （Fig. 1-07）：The liver is enlarged, the capsule is tight, and the cut surface of the liver is gray and cloudy swelling.

2. 脂肪变性 Fatty change（steatosis）

肝脂肪变性（图 1-08）：小儿肝脏体积略增大，表面及切面均呈淡黄色，切面较钝，切面有油腻的外观。

Hepatic steatosis （Fig. 1-08）：The kid's liver is slightly enlarged, the surface and the cut surface are light yellow, the edges are round and blunt, and the cut surface has a greasy appearance.

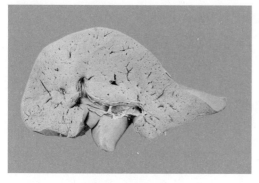

图 1-07　肝细胞水肿

Fig. 1-07　Hepatocyte edema

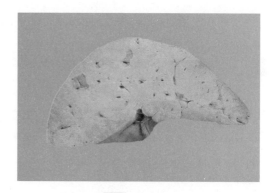

图 1-08　肝脂肪变性

Fig. 1-08　Hepatic steatosis

3. 玻璃样变性 Hyaline degeneration

脾包膜玻璃样变（图 1-09）：局部脾包膜比正常包膜明显增厚（➡），呈灰白色、半透明、均匀一致的毛玻璃样物质（★）。

思考：本病变属于何种玻璃样变性？

Hyaline degeneration of splenic capsule （Fig. 1-09）：Some of the splenic capsules are significantly thicker than the normal capsule （➡）, showing gray-white, translucent, uniform ground glass-like substances （★）.

Question：What kind of hyaline degeneration does this lesion belong to?

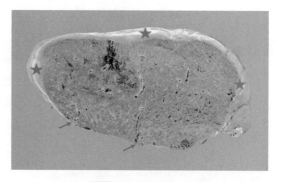

图 1-09　脾包膜玻璃样变

Fig. 1-09　Hyaline degeneration of splenic capsule

4. **病理性色素沉着 Pathological pigmentation**

（1）黑色素：黑色素瘤，肿瘤因黑色素沉积呈黑色。具体标本见本书第五章（肿瘤）。

Melanin：Melanoma, the tumor is black due to melanin deposition. The specimens can be found in Chapter 5（Tumors）.

（2）含铁血黄素：慢性肺淤血时，肺组织因含铁血黄素沉着，局灶呈棕黄色。具体标本见本书第三章（局部血液循环障碍）。

Hemosiderin：When chronic pulmonary congestion occurs, the lung tissue is yellow-stained due to irony blood, and the focal area is brownish-yellow. The specimens can be found in Chapter 3（Local Hemodynamic Disorders）.

（三）不可逆性损伤——坏死 Irreversible injury—necrosis

1. 凝固性坏死 Coagulative necrosis

（1）脾凝固性坏死（图 1-10）：脾脏局部见灰白色、质实、略呈颗粒状的三角形病灶（凝固性坏死）（★），坏死病灶周围被灰白色致密组织包围（➡）。

Coagulative necrosis of the spleen（Fig. 1-10）：The spleen has a triangular grayish-white solid granule-like lesion（coagulative necrosis）（★）surrounded by grayish-white dense tissue（➡）.

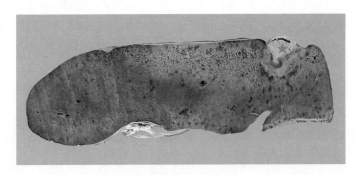

图 1-10　脾凝固性坏死
Fig. 1-10　Coagulative necrosis of the spleen

（2）肾凝固性坏死（图 1-11）：病变肾脏中可见一个质实、略呈颗粒状的灰白色病灶（凝固性坏死）（★）。

Renal coagulative necrosis（Fig. 1-11）：There is a grayish-white lesion with the slightly granular appearance（coagulative necrosis）（★）.

2. 液化性坏死 Liquefactive necrosis

（1）脑液化性坏死（图 1-12）：脑冠状切面，局部脑组织可见液化性坏死灶，灰质与白质分界不清，疏松，部分有小囊腔（★）形成。

思考：液化性坏死与凝固性坏死有什么不同？

Cerebral liquefactive necrosis （Fig. 1-12）：Coronal section of the brain, liquefactive necrosis in the local brain tissue, unclear boundary between gray matter and white matter, loose, and some small cysts （★）formed.

Question：What is the difference between liquefactive necrosis and coagulative necrosis?

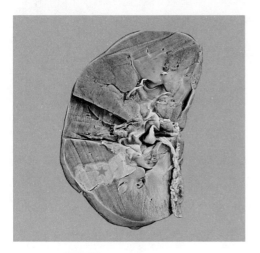

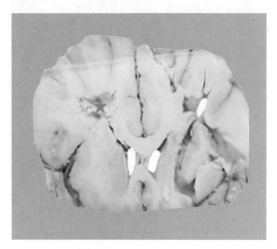

图 1-11　肾凝固性坏死

Fig. 1-11　Renal coagulative necrosis

图 1-12　脑液化性坏死

Fig. 1-12　Cerebral liquefactive necrosis

（2）肺脓肿：局部肺组织已发生坏死，坏死组织呈液状，部分液体已经流失，局部可见空腔形成。具体标本参见本书第四章（炎症）。

Pulmonary abscess：Necrosis has occurred in the local lung tissue, the necrotic tissue is liquid, some of the fluid has been lost, and the cavity is formed locally. For specific specimens, see Chapter 4 （Inflammation）.

（3）阿米巴肝脓肿（图 1-13）：肝脏局部组织明显坏死，形成含有"脓液"的腔。请注意该脓肿与肺脓肿的发生机制不同。

Amoebic abscess of the liver （Figure 1-13）：The local tissue of the liver is obviously necrotic, forming a cavity containing "pus". Please note that this abscess is different from the lung abscess.

3. 干酪样坏死 Caseous necrosis

淋巴结结核（图 1-14）：淋巴结切面有灰黄色（标本经福尔马林固定后呈灰白色）、均质、细腻的坏死灶，类似乳酪或豆腐乳的切面。

Lymph node tuberculosis （Fig. 1-14）：The section of lymph node is grayish-yellow （the specimen is grayish-white after formalin fixation）, homogeneous and delicate necrotic foci, which resembles the section of cheese or fermented bean curd.

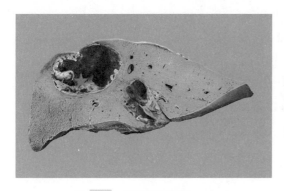

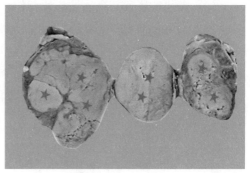

图 1-13　阿米巴肝脓肿

Fig. 1-13　Amoebic abscess of the liver

图 1-14　淋巴结结核

Fig. 1-14　Lymph node tuberculosis

4. 坏疽 Gangrene

足干性坏疽（图 1-15）：手术截肢标本，下肢末端脚趾干硬、皱缩，呈黑色（★），与周围正常组织分界清楚（➡）。

Foot dry gangrene （Fig. 1-15）：Surgical amputation specimens, the toes of the lower extremities are hard and wrinkled black（★）, with clear demarcation from surrounding normal tissues （➡）.

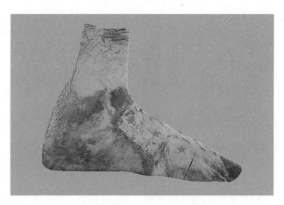

图 1-15　足干性坏疽

Fig. 1-15　Foot dry gangrene

三、 组织切片观察 Observation of tissue slides

（一）适应 Adaptation

1. 萎缩 Atrophy

心肌细胞萎缩（图 1-16）：心肌细胞比正常细胞体积缩小（★），细胞质中可见棕黄色色素颗粒(脂褐素)(➡)。

Cardiomyocyte atrophy(Fig. 1-16)：Cardiomyocyte cells are smaller(★) than normal cells, and brown pigment particle(lipofuscin)(➡)are seen in the cytoplasm.

2. 增生 Proliferation

前列腺增生症：前列腺组织中腺体、纤维及平滑肌均发生增生。具体组织切片观察见第十一章(生殖系统疾病与乳腺疾病)。

Benign prostatic hyperplasia：Prostate tissue glands, fibers and smooth muscle are hyperplastic. See Chapter 11 (Diseases of the Genital System and the Breast).

3. 肥大和增生 Hypertrophy and hyperplasia

毒性甲状腺肿组织中,滤泡上皮细胞增生,体积增大。具体组织切片观察见第十二章(内分泌系统疾病)。

In toxic goiter, follicular epithelial cells proliferate and increase in volume. See Chapter 12 (Diseases of the Endocrine System).

4. 化生 Metaplasia

肠上皮化生(图 1-17)：慢性萎缩性胃炎组织中,胃黏膜变薄,正常腺体减少和缩小(★),黏膜上皮被肠上皮[杯状细胞(➡)、潘氏细胞或吸收上皮]所取代。

思考：什么组织发生了萎缩?

Intestinal metaplasia(Fig. 1-17)：In chronic atrophic gastritis, gastric mucosa becomes thin, the gastric mucosal epithelia are replaced by intestinal epithelium [goblet cells(➡), some Paneth's cells or absorbing epithelium].

Question：Which tissue is atrophied?

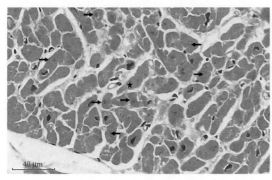 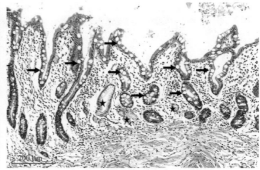

图 1-16　心肌细胞萎缩　　　　　图 1-17　肠上皮化生
Fig. 1-16　Cardiomyocte atrophy　　　Fig. 1-17　Intestinal metaplasia

（二）可逆性损伤——变性 Reversible injury—degeneration

1. 细胞水肿(水变性)Cellular swelling (Hydropic degeneration)

（1）肾脏细胞水肿（图 1-18）：病变主要分布在皮质区肾小球（★）周围的近曲小管（➡），远曲小管（▲）病变不明显。近曲小管上皮体积增大，胞浆内有多数红染的细颗粒（➤）。

思考：为什么细胞水肿主要发生在近曲小管上皮细胞？

Renal cell swelling (Fig. 1-18): The lesions are mainly distributed in the proximal convoluted tubule (➡) around the glomerular (★), but not obvious in the distal convoluted tubule (▲). The volume of proximal convoluted tubule epithelium increases, and there are many red-stained granules in the cytoplasm.

Question: Why does it mainly occur in proximal convoluted tubular epithelial cells?

（2）肝细胞水肿（图 1-19）：肝细胞体积明显增大，大小不等，部分细胞呈球状增大。肝细胞胞浆疏松，呈颗粒状（★），部分透明呈空泡状，为气球样变；肝窦扭曲、狭窄、闭塞（➡）。

Hepatocyte edema (Fig. 1-19): The volume of hepatocytes is obviously increased, with variable size and some were spherically enlarged. The cytoplasm of hepatocytes was loose and granular (★), with some transparent and vacuolar, which is a balloon-like change. The sinuses of the liver were twisted, narrowed and occluded (➡).

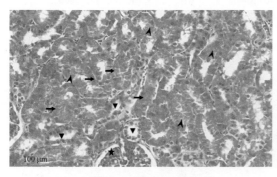

图 1-18　肾脏细胞水肿
Fig. 1-18　Renal cell swelling

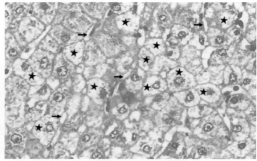

图 1-19　肝细胞水肿
Fig. 1-19　Hepatocyte edema

2. 脂肪变性 Fatty change(Steatosis)

（1）肝脂肪变性（图 1-20）：脂肪变性的肝细胞体积增大，肝细胞核周可见许多大小不等的空泡（➡），甚至空泡融合变大，充满胞浆，将细胞核挤向边缘，以致与脂肪细胞相似。肝窦狭窄。

思考：如何证实肝细胞内的空泡为脂滴？

Hepatic steatosis（Fig. 1-20）: In fatty degeneration of the cells, there is an increase of the size, there are many vacuoles of different sizes（➡️）in the cytoplasm around the nucleus, and some coalesce to form one large vacuole filling the cell, displacing the nucleus to the periphery of the cell, so that they are similar to adipocytes. The sinusoids become narrow.

Question: How to confirm that the vacuoles in the liver cells are lipid droplets?

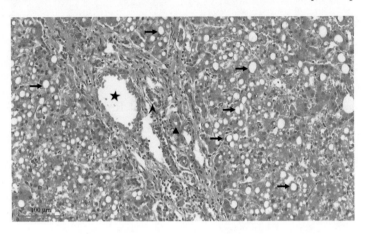

★ :小叶间静脉 interlobular vein; ▲ :小叶间动脉 interlobular artery;
➤ :小叶间胆管 interlobular bile duct.

图 1-20　肝脂肪变性

Fig. 1-20　Hepatic steatosis

3. 玻璃样变 Hyaline degeneration

（1）肾小管上皮细胞内玻璃样变（图 1-21）:肾近曲小管上皮细胞内可见均质红染的圆形小体（➡️）。

Intracellular hyaline degeneration of the renal tubular epithelial cells（Fig. 1-21）: Homogeneous red-stained round bodies（➡️）were seen in renal proximal convoluted tubular epithelial cells.

（2）纤维结缔组织玻璃样变（图 1-22）:为疤痕组织,胶原纤维平行或交错分布;纤维细胞稀少,小血管稀少;胶原纤维增粗,相互融合成均质、红染物质。

Hyaline degeneration of the connective tissue（Fig. 1-22）: It is a scar tissue. Collagen fibrils distribute in a parallel or cross mode. Fibrocytes and small vessels are sparse. Dense collagenous fibrils assume a homogeneous pink hyaline appearance.

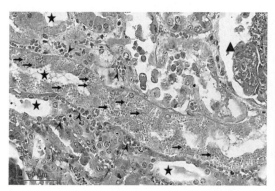

★:肾小管腔 renal tubular lumen；▲:肾小球 glomerulus；
◣:血管内红细胞 intravascular red blood cells.

图 1-21 肾小管上皮细胞内玻璃样变

Fig. 1-21 Intracellular hyaline degeneration of
the renal tubular epithelial cells

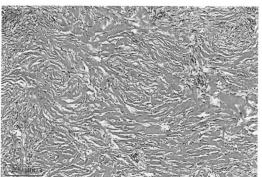

图 1-22 纤维结缔组织玻璃样变

Fig. 1-22 Hyaline degeneration of the
connective tissue

（3）脾中央动脉玻璃样变（图 1-23）:脾脏白髓（★）中的中央动脉（➡）管壁增厚,呈均质红染的无细胞结构状态,管腔狭窄。

Hyaline degeneration of the central artery of the spleen（Fig. 1-23）:The wall of the central artery（➡）in the white pulp（★）of the spleen is thickened, showing a homogeneous red stained acellular structure with a narrow lumen.

4. 病理性色素沉着 Pathological pigmentation

（1）含铁血黄素（图 1-24）:吞噬细胞内充满大小不一的棕褐色细颗粒状色素。

思考:如何证实棕褐色色素颗粒是含铁血黄素?

Hemosiderin（Fig 1-24）: The phagocytic cells are filled with tan, finely granular hemosiderin pigments of varying size.

Question: How to confirm that the brown pigment particles are hemosiderin?

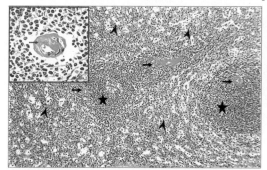

★: 白髓 the white pulp；◣: 红髓 the red pulp；
➡: 中央动脉 the central artery.

图 1-23 脾中央动脉玻璃样变

Fig. 1-23 Hyaline degeneration of the central
artery of the spleen

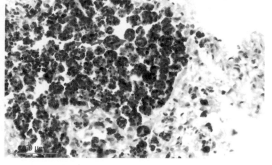

图 1-24 含铁血黄素

Fig. 1-24 Hemosiderin

（2）脂褐素：见本章心肌细胞萎缩（图1-16）。

Lipofuscin：See cardiomyocyte atrophy in this chapter（Fig. 1-16）.

5. 病理性钙化 Pathologic calcification

组织切片观察见本章肺干酪样坏死伴钙化。

See pulmonary caseous necrosis with calcification of this chapter.

（三）不可逆性损伤——坏死 Irreversible injury—necrosis

1. 凝固性坏死 Coagulative necrosis

（1）肾凝固性坏死（图1-25）：与正常肾小球（★）及肾小管（◀）相比，凝固性坏死区肾小管（▲）、肾小球（➡）等肾组织结构轮廓尚可辨认，但细胞微细结构消失，细胞核碎裂、固缩或消失，胞浆红染。

Renal coagulative necrosis（Fig. 1-25）：Coagulative necrotic areas，renal tubules（▲），glomeruli（➡）and other renal tissue structures are still identifiable by comparing with normal glomeruli（★）and tubules（◀）. However，the cellular fine structure disappeared. The necrotic cell presents karyorrhexis，pyknosis and karyolysis，and the cytoplasm shows increased eosinophilia。

2. 液化性坏死 Liquefactive necrosis

（1）脑液化性坏死（乙型脑炎）（图1-26）：脑组织（▲）内有散在大小不等、淡染、质地疏松呈网状的椭圆形软化灶（★）；软化灶内有坏死的细胞碎屑。

Cerebral liquefactive necrosis（encephalitis B）（Fig. 1-26）：There are scattered softening lesions in the brain tissue（▲），with varying sizes，light-stained，oval-shaped and loose texture（★）. There are necrotic cell debris in the softening lesions.

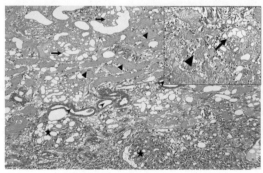
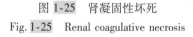
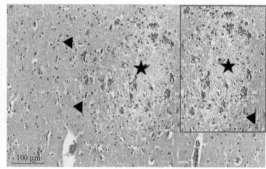

图 1-25　肾凝固性坏死　　　　　　　图 1-26　脑液化性坏死（乙型脑炎）
Fig. 1-25　Renal coagulative necrosis　　　Fig. 1-26　Cerebral liquefactive necrosis（encephalitis B）

（2）肺脓肿：局部正常肺组织结构消失，代之以大量中性粒细胞浸润。组织切片观察见第四章（炎症）。

思考：导致液化性坏死的机制是什么？

Pulmonary abscess：The local normal lung tissue structure disappeared and are replaced by a large number of neutrophil infiltrations. See Chapter 4 (Inflammation).

Question：What is the mechanism that leads to liquefactive necrosis?

3. 纤维素样坏死 Fibrinoid necrosis

血管壁纤维素样坏死（图1-27）：某些类型的肾小球肾炎病变中，肾小球入球小动脉（➡）和肾小球毛细血管壁（◀）发生纤维素样坏死，血管壁呈红染的颗粒状或条块状结构。

Fibrinoid necrosis of the vessel wall （Fig. 1-27）：In some types of glomerulonephritis, glomerular small arteries （➡） and glomerular capillary wall （◀） undergo fibrinoid necrosis, and the vascular walls are red-stained granular or strip-like structures.

4. 干酪样坏死 Caseous necrosis

（1）淋巴结干酪样坏死（图1-28）：局部淋巴结正常结构（▲）消失，被大量红染、无结构的颗粒状物（★）取代。组织坏死彻底，未见原来的组织结构，核碎片少见。

Caseous necrosis of lymph nodes （Fig. 1-28）：The normal structure of local lymph nodes （▲） disappeared, replaced by a large number of red-stained, unstructured granules （★）. The tissue necrosis was complete, without the original tissue structure, and the nuclear debris is rare.

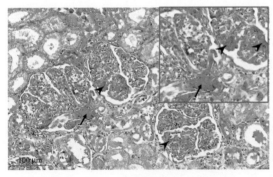
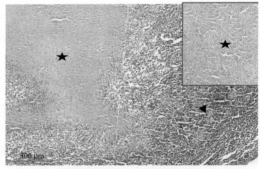

图 1-27 血管壁纤维素样坏死   图 1-28 淋巴结干酪样坏死

Fig. 1-27 Fibrinoid necrosis of the vessel wall   Fig. 1-28 Caseous necrosis of lymph nodes

（2）肺干酪样坏死伴钙化（图1-29）：肺结核干酪样坏死病灶在镜下为红染无结构的颗粒状物（★）；周边纤维组织（➡）增生包裹，继而坏死物逐渐干燥浓缩，并有钙盐（▲）沉着。

思考：坏死组织有哪些结局？本例切片中你看到了哪些坏死的结局？

Pulmonary caseous necrosis with calcification （Fig. 1-29）：Caseous necrosis of tuberculosis with red-stained, unstructured granules（★）（under the microscope）; surrounding fibrous tissue （➡） proliferated and wrapped, and then the necrosis gradually dried and concentrated, with calcium salts （▲） deposited.

Question：What are the outcomes of necrotic tissue? What necrotic outcomes did you see in this slides?

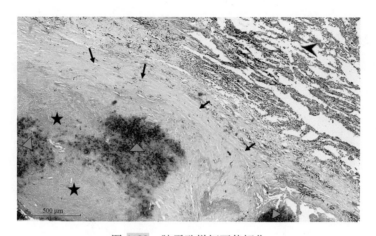

图 1-29   肺干酪样坏死伴钙化

Fig. 1-29   Pulmonary caseous necrosis with calcification

四、 病例讨论 Case discussion

患者，女，50 岁，有糖尿病病史 10 年。最近发现左侧下肢高度肿胀、发黑，病变组织与正常组织之间的分界不清。

The patient, a 50-year-old woman, had a history of diabetes for 10 years. Recently, it was found that the left lower extremity was highly swollen and black. The demarcation between the diseased tissue and the normal tissue is not clear.

思考：该患者下肢发生了何种病变？为什么？

Question：What kind of pathological changes occur in the lower limbs of this patient? Why?

五、 思考题 Questions

（1）萎缩的概念是什么？导致萎缩的常见原因有哪些？

What is the concept of atrophy? What are the common causes of atrophy?

（2）何谓化生？化生有哪些类型，有何临床意义？

What is metaplasia? What types are there? What is the clinical significance?

（3）何谓病理性钙化？其常见类型的异同点有哪些？

What is pathological calcification? What are the similarities and differences between their common types?

（4）坏死的基本病变有哪些？其常见类型有哪些？

What are the basic pathological changes of necrosis? What are the common types?

（5）什么是坏疽？三种坏疽的区别有什么不同？

What is gangrene? What are the differences between the three types of gangrene?

编写 Written by：邓敏 Deng Min

英文审校 English proofreader：刘瑶 Liu Yao

2

第二章　损伤的修复

Chapter 2　Tissue Repair

一、　教学目的 Teaching objectives

（1）掌握创伤愈合的过程及各种组织的再生能力。

Master the wound healing process and the regeneration capacity of various tissues.

（2）掌握肉芽组织的形态特点及其在组织修复中的意义。

Master the morphological characteristics of granulation tissues and its significance in tissue repair.

二、　大体标本观察 Observation of gross specimens

（1）皮肤疤痕（图2-01）：皮肤组织中央可见一条略隆起于表面的疤痕（➡），疤痕颜色较为灰白。

思考:这种疤痕组织属于一期愈合还是二期愈合？

Skin scar（Fig. 2-01）：A scar（➡）slightly protruding from the surface of the skin is visible in the center of the skin. The scar is grayish.

Question：Does this scar tissue belong to the first stage of healing or the second stage of healing?

（2）创伤性神经瘤（图2-02）：一段坐骨神经（➡）的一端粗细均匀,神经束走向一致;另一端膨大成瘤状物（★）。

Traumatic neuroma（Fig. 2-02）：This is a segment of sciatic nerve（➡）, with one end of the uniform thickness and the same extending direction, and the other end expanding into a tumor（★）.

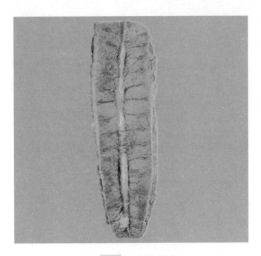

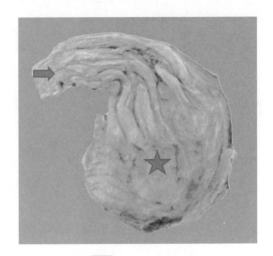

图 2-01　皮肤疤痕

Fig. 2-01　Skin scar

图 2-02　创伤性神经瘤

Fig. 2-02　Traumatic neuroma

（3）骨折愈合（图 2-03）：骨折处有梭形骨痂形成（➡），左侧为正常骨。

思考：骨折愈合分几个阶段？影响骨折愈合的因素有哪些？

Fracture healing（Fig. 2-03）：There is a spindle-shaped bony callus at the fracture site. The left side is a normal bone.

Question：How many stages of fracture healing are there? What are the factors that affect fracture healing?

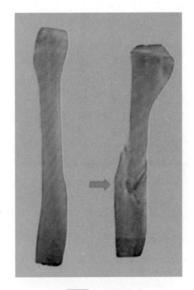

图 2-03　骨折愈合

Fig. 2-03　Fracture healing

三、 组织切片观察 Observation of tissue slides

（1）肝细胞再生（图2-04）：亚急性重症肝炎时，残留肝细胞呈结节状再生（★），肝细胞再生结节之间为坏死的肝组织（➡）。

思考：根据再生能力分类，肝细胞属于哪类细胞？ 本例病变属于完全性再生吗？

Hepatocytes regeneration（Fig. 2-04）: In the case of subacute severe hepatitis, residual hepatocytes are regenerated in nodules（★）, and hepatocytes between the nodules are necrotic（➡）.

Question: According to the classification of regenerative capacity, what kind of cells does hepatocytes belong to? Is this lesion a complete regeneration?

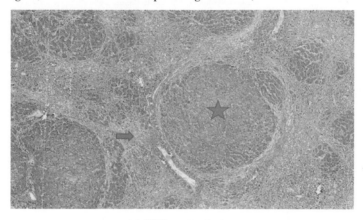

图 2-04   肝细胞再生

Fig. 2-04   Hepatocytes regeneration

（2）肉芽组织（图2-05）：局部正常的鳞状上皮消失，组织缺失处可见大量平行排列的、与创面垂直的新生毛细血管（➡）。毛细血管间组织水肿、疏松，其中可见成纤维细胞（▲）及炎细胞浸润（◤）。肉芽组织下方为成熟的纤维组织，血管减少，炎细胞消失，成纤维细胞产生大量胶原纤维并继发玻璃样变，最后转化为瘢痕组织。

思考：创伤愈合的影响因素有哪些？

Granulation tissue（Fig. 2-05）: The local normal squamous epithelium disappeared, and a large number of parallel-arranged new capillaries（➡）perpendicular to the wound surface are observed in the tissue loss. The inter-capillary tissue showed edema and looseness, and among them, there are fibroblasts（▲）and inflammatory cells infiltration（◤）. Under the granulation tissue is mature fibrotic tissue. Where the blood vessels are reduced, the inflammatory cells disappear and the fibroblasts produce a large amount of collagen fibers and undergo a glassy change, which would finally become scar tissue.

Question：What are the factors that affect the wound healing?

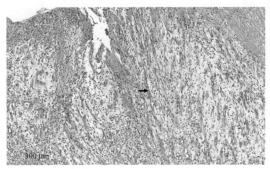 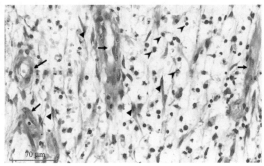

低倍镜 lower magnification　　　　　　　　高倍镜 higher magnification

图 2-05　肉芽组织

Fig. 2-05　Granulation tissue

四、 病例讨论 Case discussion

1963 年 1 月,患者王某,右前臂被冲床轧断。在医务人员的努力下,患者的断臂再植成功,断肢功能基本恢复。这是我国第一例断肢再植成功病例。

请思考:断肢再植中有哪些组织发生了创伤愈合? 其愈合的过程如何?

In January 1963, the patient Wang, his right forearm was cut off by the punching machine. After the efforts of medical staff, the replantation was successful and the limb function was basically restored. This was the first successful replantation case of the broken limb in China.

Question：Which tissues in the replantation of the limbs have healed? What is the healing process?

五、 思考题 Questions

(1) 根据再生能力,机体的细胞分为哪几类细胞? 其临床意义是什么?

According to the ability to regenerate, what types of cells are the body cells divided into? What is the corresponding clinical significance?

(2) 何谓肉芽组织? 请描述其形态结构和主要功能。

What is the the granulation tissue? Please describe its morphological structure and main function.

(3) 何为创伤愈合? 一期愈合和二期愈合的区别有哪些?

What is the wound healing? What are the differences between primary healing and secondary healing?

编写 Written by：董亮 Dong Liang
中文审校 Chinese proofreader：邓敏 Deng Min
英文审校 English proofreader：刘瑶 Liu Yao

3

第三章　局部血液循环障碍

Chapter 3　Local Hemodynamic Disorder

一、　教学目的 Teaching Objectives

（1）掌握肺和肝慢性淤血的形态特点及后果。

Master the morphological characteristics and consequences of chronic congestion of lung and liver.

（2）熟悉出血的原因及后果。

Be familiar with the causes and consequences of hemorrhage.

（3）掌握血栓形成的条件、形态特点、结局及其对机体的影响。

Master the conditions, morphological characteristics, outcomes of thrombosis and its effects on the body.

（4）熟悉主要脏器梗死的发生原因、形态特点及后果。

Be familiar with the causes, morphological characteristics and consequences of major organ infarction.

二、　大体标本观察 Observation of gross specimens

（一）淤血 Congestion

（1）慢性肝淤血（图3-01）：肝淤血时,体积增大,包膜紧张、光滑,表面（图3-01a）及切面（图3-01b）呈暗红色与黄色相间的网状结构（➡）,形如中药槟榔的剖面,故称之为槟榔肝。肝小叶中央区因淤血严重,中央静脉及肝窦扩张呈红色;肝小叶周边区的肝细胞发生脂肪变性,呈黄色。

Chronic hepatic congestion（Fig. 3-01）：When hepatic congestion occurs, the liver is enlarged with tight and smooth capsule, the surface（Fig. 3-01a）and cut surface（Fig. 3-01b）has a dark red and yellow appearance（➡）, similar to traditional Chinese medicine *Areca catechu*. The appearance of such congested liver is called "nutmeg liver". In the central area of the hepatic lobules, which were red, the central vein and hepatic sinus were dilated due to congestion. While the hepatocytes in the peripheral area of the hepatic lobules were yellowish due to fatty degeneration.

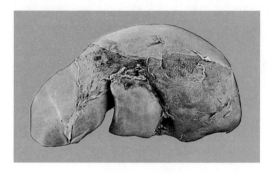
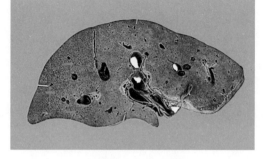

a. 表面 the surface   b. 切面 the cut surface

Fig.3-01   慢性肝淤血

Fig.3-01   Chronic hepatic congestion

（2）慢性肺淤血（图 3-02）：在胸膜下及肺切面均可见到散在的黑色或棕色斑点（➡）。切面观，褐色肺组织比正常肺组织更致密，质地更硬；慢性肺淤血导致红细胞漏出到肺泡腔内，然后被巨噬细胞吞噬，吞噬细胞内的血红蛋白降解并形成含铁血黄素。有时，充血伴随着肺泡壁纤维组织的增殖，导致"肺部褐色硬化"。

Chronic pulmonary congestion(Fig. 3-02)：Some black or brown spots（➡）can be seen in the subpleural and lung sections. On cut surface, the brownish congested lungs are firmer and denser than normal lungs. In case of chronic pulmonary congestion, the erythrocytes leak into alveolar cavities and then, they are engulfed by macrophages. Hemosiderin is formed after breaking of hemoglobin within the phagocytes. Sometimes the congestion is accompanied with the proliferation of fibrous tissue of alveolar walls, resulting in "brown induration of lung".

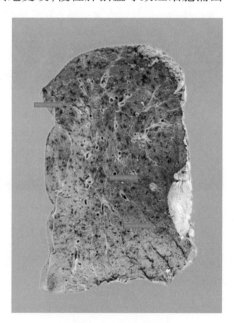

图 3-02   慢性肺淤血

Fig.3-02   Chronic pulmonary congestion

（二）血栓形成 Thrombosis

（1）门静脉血栓（图3-03）：图3-03a 为肝内门静脉纵剖面，其主要分支的管腔被一条棕褐色/灰黄色的新鲜血栓充满（➡）。图3-03b 为肝内门静脉分支横断面（➡），可见腔内充满灰黄色与棕褐色相间的血栓，血管壁明显增厚。两图均为血吸虫病肝硬化标本。

思考题：血栓形成的可能因素有哪些？

Portal vein thrombosis（Fig. 3-03）：Fig. 3-03a is a longitudinal section of the intrahepatic portal vein, in which the lumen of the main branch is filled with a sepia/gray-yellow fresh thrombus（➡）. Fig. 3-03b shows the cross section of the intrahepatic portal vein branch（➡）. It can be seen that the cavity is filled with gray-yellow and tan-colored thrombus, and the vessel wall is obviously thickened. Both samples were schistosomiasis cirrhosis.

Question：What are the possible factors for thrombosis?

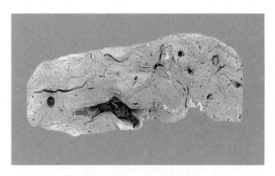 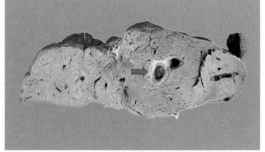

a. 纵切面 longitudinal section　　　　b. 横切面 transverse section

图 3-03　门静脉血栓

Fig. 3-03　Portal vein thrombosis

（2）股动脉血栓（图3-04）：一段已被剪开的股动脉及其分支，动脉腔内有一棕褐色与灰黄色相间的长长的马鞍状血栓（➡）。

Femoral artery thrombosis（Fig. 3-04）：The femoral artery and its bifurcation have been opened to reveal a long saddle embolus（➡）with apparent laminations alternating with dark brown layers and gray-yellow layers.

（3）主动脉动脉瘤内血栓（图3-05）：主动脉内膜粗糙，主动脉弓部管壁向外膨出形成所谓动脉瘤，其内壁附有棕褐色血栓（➡）。此例动脉瘤为梅毒性主动脉炎的后果，这是因为梅毒性病变破坏了主动脉的中层弹力纤维，造成该处管壁抵抗力薄弱，在动脉血流的压力下向外膨出形成瘤样外观，因此它并非真性肿瘤。

思考题：为什么在此动脉瘤内会有血栓形成？血栓形成可能有什么后果？

Aortic aneurysm thrombosis（Fig. 3-05）：The aortic intima is rough, and the aortic arch wall bulges outward to form a so-called aneurysm with a brown thrombus（➡）on its inner wall.

This aneurysm is a consequence of syphilitic aortitis. This is because the syphilitic lesion destroys the middle layer of elastic fibers of the aorta, resulting in weak resistance of the wall and bulging out under the pressure of arterial blood flow, so it is not a true tumor.

　　Question: Why is there thrombosis in this aneurysm? What are the possible consequences?

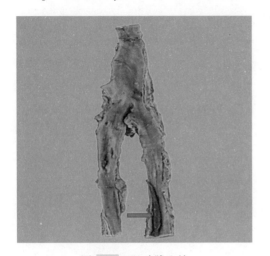

图 3-04　股动脉血栓
Fig. 3-04　Femoral artery thrombosis

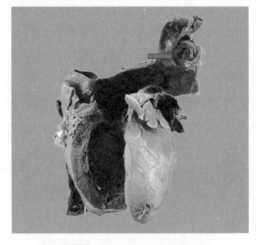

图 3-05　主动脉动脉瘤内血栓
Fig. 3-05　Aortic aneurysm thrombosis

　　(4) 左心房附壁血栓(图 3-06): 左心房明显扩大,左心房壁上有一不规则球形血栓(➡)。血栓呈灰褐色,与心内膜紧密连接。

　　Mural thrombus in the left atrium (Fig. 3-06): The left atrium is obviously enlarged and an irregular globular thrombus (➡) can be seen in the cardiac cavity of left atrium. It is gray-brown and adhered tightly to the endocardium.

　　此例患者患风湿性心脏病,死亡前一周曾发生频繁的心房纤维颤动(心房发生快而细的乱颤,每分钟可达 400~600 次)。

　　思考题:此例心房附壁血栓发生的因素是什么? 可能产生什么后果?

　　The patient suffered from rheumatic heart disease. Frequent atrial fibrillation (rapid and fine atrial fibrillation, up to 400 – 600 times per minute) occurred one week before death.

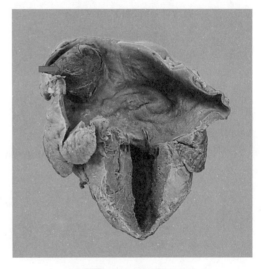

图 3-06　左心房附壁血栓
Fig. 3-06　Mural thrombus in the left atrium

　　Question: What are the causes of atrial mural thrombosis in this case? What are the possible consequences?

（三）出血 Hemorrhage

（1）大脑出血（图 3-07）：大脑内囊有不规则大块黑色出血灶（➡），造成脑组织破坏。本例是高血压病所致。

Cerebral hemorrhage（Fig. 3-07）：There is an irregularly hemorrhagic focus（➡）in the inner capsule of the brain causing brain tissue destruction. This case is caused by hypertension.

（2）脾出血（图 3-08）：脾实质内可见大块黑色出血灶（➡）。该患者是从高处跌落导致脾破裂。

Splenic hemorrhage（Fig. 3-08）：There is a large hemorrhagic foci（➡）in the splenic parenchyma. The patient fell from a height and caused the rupture of the spleen.

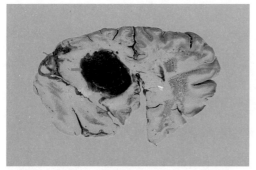

图 3-07　大脑出血
Fig. 3-07　Cerebral hemorrhage

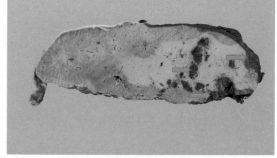

图 3-08　脾出血
Fig. 3-08　Splenic hemorrhage

（3）肾出血（图 3-09）：肾髓质高度充血并出血（➡）。患者患有流行性出血热（一种急性传染病）。

Renal hemorrhage（Fig. 3-09）：Renal medulla is highly congested and hemorrhagic（➡）. The patient has epidemic hemorrhagic fever（an acute infectious disease）.

思考题：上述各种标本中出血原因是什么？出血对机体有何影响？

Question ：What is the cause of hemorrhage in the above-mentioned specimens? What is the impact on the body?

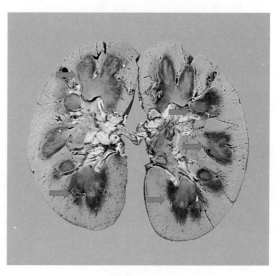

图 3-09　肾出血
Fig. 3-09　Renal hemorrhage

（四）梗死 Infarction

1. 贫血性梗死 Anemic infarction

（1）心肌梗死：病变描述见第六章（心血管系统疾病）。

Myocardial infarction：The lesion will be described in Chapter 6（Diseases of the Heart and Blood Vessels System）.

（2）脾贫血性梗死（图3-10）：图3-10a为较新鲜的梗死，脾脏切面可见分界明显的楔形梗死灶（➡），底朝向脾包膜，尖端朝向脾门。梗死灶表面隆起，切面苍白、干燥，梗死边缘已开始机化。图3-10b为较陈旧的梗死，梗死区由结缔组织所代替，之后因疤痕收缩而凹陷（➡）。

Anemic infarcts of the spleen（Fig. 3-10）：Figure 3-10a shows a fresher infarction. The spleen section shows a wedge-shaped infarct（➡）with a clear boundary. The bottom is toward the spleen capsule and the tip is toward the spleen. The surface of the infarct was raised, the section was pale and dry, and the infarct edge began to be organized. Figure 3-10b shows the older infarction. The infarct area is replaced by connective tissue, and the scar is contracted later（➡）.

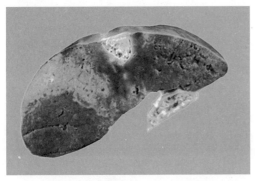 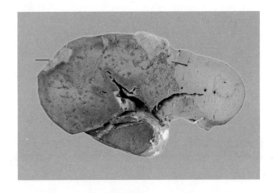

a. 新鲜脾梗死 fresher infarction   b. 陈旧脾梗死 older infarction

图 3-10　脾贫血性梗死

Fig. 3-10　Anemic infarcts of the spleen

（3）肾贫血性梗死（图3-11）：梗死灶呈黄白色、境界分明的楔状（➡），底朝向肾包膜，尖端朝向肾门。

Anemic infarct of the kidney（Fig. 3-11）：The infarct is yellow-white, with a well-defined wedge（➡）, with the bottom facing the renal capsule and the tip facing the renal hilum.

（4）脑梗死（图3-12）：在大脑剖面，脑组织有大片不规则的软化坏死区，此处正常结构被破坏，质地疏松呈糨糊状。

Infarct of the brain（Fig. 3-12）：In the brain section, there are large areas of irregular softening and necrosis in the brain tissue, where the normal structure is destroyed and the texture is loose and paste-like.

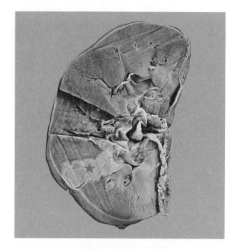

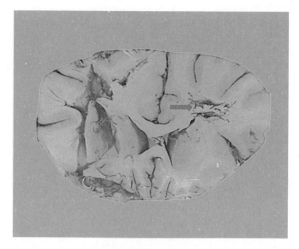

图 3-11　肾贫血性梗死

Fig. 3-11　Anemic infarct of the kidney

图 3-12　脑梗死

Fig. 3-12　Infarct of the brain

2. 出血性梗死 Hemorrhagic infarction

（1）肠出血性梗死（图 3-13）：梗死肠浆膜面失去光泽，呈灰褐黑色。肠壁增厚，肠壁各层均可见出血、坏死。

Hemorrhagic infarct of the intestine (Fig. 3-13): The infarcted serosal membrane surface loses luster and is grayish brownish black. The intestinal wall is thickened, and all layers of the intestinal wall are hemorrhagic and necrotic.

（2）肺出血性梗死（图 3-14）：肺出血梗死区邻近包膜下，呈楔形，暗红或灰黑色，正常肺泡结构不清。

Hemorrhagic infarct of the lung (Fig. 3-14): The pulmonary hemorrhagic infarct area is close to the capsule, showing a wedge shape, dark red or grayish black, and the normal alveolar structure is unclear.

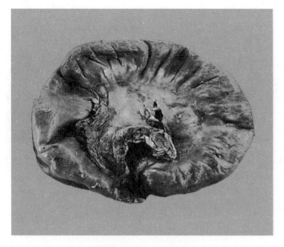

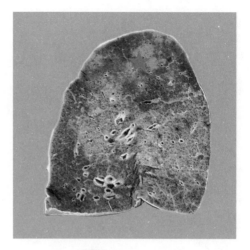

图 3-13 肠出血性梗死

Fig. 3-13 Hemorrhagic infarct of the intestine

图 3-14 肺出血性梗死

Fig. 3-14 Hemorrhagic infarct of the lung

三、组织切片观察 Observation of tissue slides

(一) 淤血 Congestion

(1) 肺淤血(图3-15):急性肺淤血时(图3-15a),肺泡壁毛细血管扩张、充血(➡)。肺泡腔内见淡红色漏出液(▲),并见少量漏出的红细胞。慢性肺淤血时(图3-15b),肺泡间隔增厚、纤维组织增多(✈),肺泡腔或肺泡间隔可见大量吞噬了含铁血黄素的巨噬细胞(被称为"心衰细胞")(★)。

Pulmonary congestion (fig. 3-15): In acute congestion (fig. 3-15a), the capillaries of the alveolar wall are dilated and congested (➡). There is reddish leaking fluid (▲) and a small amount of red blood cells in alveolar cavity. In chronic pulmonary congestion (fig. 3-15b), the septa become thickened and fibrotic (✈), and the alveolar spaces and alveolar septa contain numerous hemosiderin-laden macrophages, which are then called "heart failure cells" (★).

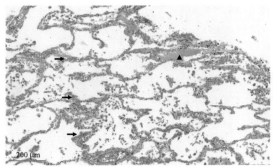

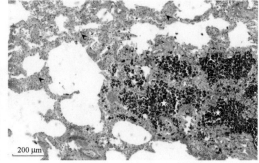

a. 急性肺淤血 acute pulmonary congestion　　　　b. 慢性肺淤血 chronic pulmonary congestion

图 3-15　肺淤血

Fig. 3-15　Pulmonary congestion

（2）慢性肝淤血（图3-16）：肝脏正常结构保留，肝小叶中央部分淤血严重；肝小叶中央静脉（★）及附近肝窦高度扩张（▲），中央静脉周围的肝窦压迫肝细胞导致肝细胞萎缩（➡），小叶周边的肝细胞相对正常（＋），部分肝细胞脂肪变性（◀）。有些相邻小叶的淤血部位互相沟通。

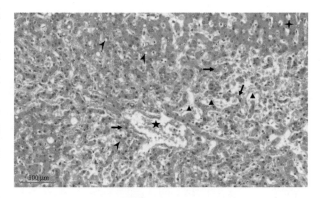

图 3-16　慢性肝淤血

Fig. 3-16　Chronic congestion of the liver

Chronic congestion of the liver (Fig. 3- 16）：The normal structure of the liver is preserved, and the central part of the hepatic lobules is severely congested; the central vein of the hepatic lobules (★) and the nearby hepatic sinus are highly dilated (▲), the hepatocytes are atrophied (➡) by the sinusoids around the central vein, and the hepatocytes around the lobules are relatively normal (＋), partial hepatic steatosis (◀). Some of the adjacent lobular confluences communicate with each other.

（二）血栓形成 Thrombus

（1）新鲜血栓（图3-17）：血栓位于静脉腔内，部分与血管壁附着。该血管壁有玻璃样变。血栓呈分层结构，其中淡粉红色细颗粒状的为血小板凝聚形成的小梁状结构（★），小梁边缘可见中性粒细胞附着（＋），小梁之间血液凝固，充满大量凝固的纤维蛋白（➡）和红细胞（◀）。此血栓为新鲜的混合血栓。

Fresh thrombus (Fig. 3- 17）：The thrombus develops in the vein and attaches to the underlying vessel wall. The vessel wall has a hyaline change. It appears apparent laminations, which are produced by pale layers of platelet（★）with numerous neutrophils（✚）attaching to their surfaces and fibrin（➡）that alternate with darker layers containing more erythrocytes（◤）. This kind of thrombus belongs to the mixed thrombus.

（2）机化血栓（图3-18）：病变在小动脉（▲为小动脉内弹力板）内，管腔内血栓已消失，为机化的纤维组织（★）及再通的血管（➡）所代替。

Organizing thrombus（Fig. 3-18）：The lesion is in a small artery（▲ a small arterial elastic plate）. The thrombus in the lumen has disappeared, and it is replaced by the proliferating connective tissue（★）and the recanalized blood vessel（➡）.

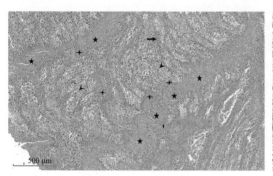

图 3-17　新鲜血栓

Fig. 3-17　Fresh thrombus

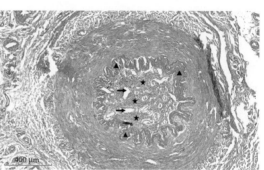

图 3-18　机化血栓

Fig. 3-18　Organizing thrombus

（三）栓塞 Embolism

（1）肺羊水栓塞（图3-19）：肺间质血管充血，多数小血管（小动脉、毛细血管）（▲）内可见呈灰红、灰蓝色的角化上皮（➡）和淡灰蓝色的黏液，肺泡内有粉红色水肿液（★）。

Amniotic liquid embolism of the lung（Fig. 3-19）：Pulmonary interstitial vascular congestion, most small blood vessels（small arteries, capillaries）（▲）can be seen in gray red/gray blue keratinized epithelium（➡）and light

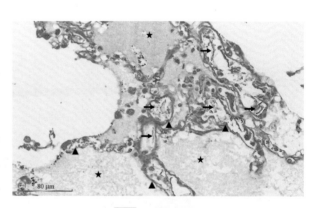

图 3-19　肺羊水栓塞

Fig. 3-19　Amniotic liquid embolism of the lung

gray blue mucus. There is pink edema（★）in the alveoli.

（2）脂肪栓塞：见本章动物实验部分。

Fat embolism：See animal experiments.

（四）梗死 Infarction

1. 贫血性梗死 Anemic infarction

（1）脾贫血性梗死（图 3-20）：先肉眼观察，多数区为不规则的楔形病灶，色较淡红。再以低倍镜从切片边缘的正常组织处向病灶处移动观察，找到梗死部位。并与周围脾组织做比较，与周围相对正常的脾组织（▲）做比较，梗死区（★）呈淡红色，细胞核均消失，但该处脾组织的轮廓仍存在。梗死区边缘充血出血带不明显。部分切片梗死区周围的红髓明显充血，白髓萎缩。

Anemic infarction of spleen（Fig. 3-20）：First naked eye observation showed that the majority of the area was an irregular wedge-shaped lesion with a pale red color. Then use a low power microscope to observe from the edge of the slides to the lesion from the normal tissue to find the infarct. Compared with the surrounding spleen tissue, compared with the normal spleen tissue（▲）, the color of the infarct area（★）is reddish and the nucleus disappears, but the contour of the spleen tissue still exists. The hemorrhagic zone at the edge of the infarcted area was not obvious. The red pulp around the infarcted area was partially congested and the white pulp was atrophied.

（2）肾贫血性梗死（图 3-21）：详细描写见第一章图 1-25。梗死灶周围组织中可见血管内的血栓（✚）及坏死组织（▲）。

Anemic infarction of kidney（Fig. 3-21）：A detailed description is shown in Figure 1-25 in Chapter 1. Intravascular thrombus（✚）and necrotic tissue（▲）in the tissue surrounding the infarct.

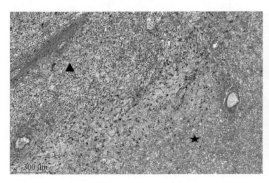

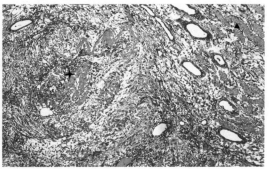

图 3-20　脾贫血性梗死

Fig. 3-20　Anemic infarction of spleen

图 3-21　肾贫血性梗死

Fig. 3-21　Anemic infarction of kidney

2. 出血性梗死 Hemorrhagic infarction

（1）肺出血性梗死（图 3-22）：肺组织局部可以见致密、红染的三角形实变区，为梗死区（★）。由于大部分细胞核消失或被出血覆盖，该区域的肺组织结构几乎消失，仅隐约可见血管及肺泡轮廓;附近肺组织淤血(▲),部分切片梗死区附近肺动脉内有血栓性栓子(◤);梗死区充满红细胞,梗死区和周围肺组织之间为充血出血带(➡)。

Hemorrhagic infarct of the lung(Fig. 3-22): A triangle shaped, dense and pink stained area is revealed in lung tissue. This is the area of hemorrhagic infarct(★) of lung tissue. Since most of the nucleus disappears or is covered by hemorrhage, the lung tissue structure of this area almost disappears, and the blood vessels and alveolar contours are faintly visible; near the infarct area pulmonary tissue congestion (▲), part of the infarct area near the pulmonary artery with thrombotic emboli (◤); infarct area filled with red blood cells, between the infarct area and surrounding lung tissue is a hyperemia and hemorrhage zone (➡).

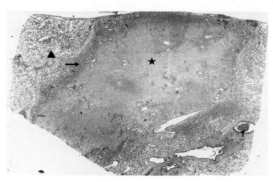 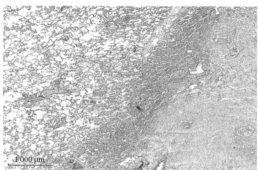

低倍镜 lower magnification　　　　　高倍镜 higher magnification

图 3-22　肺出血性梗死

Fig. 14-01　Hemorrhagic infarct of the lung

3. 败血性梗死 Septic infarction

见第十章(泌尿系统疾病)中下行性感染导致的急性肾盂肾炎的描写。

See a description of acute pyelonephritis caused by a descending infection in Chapter 10 (Diseases of the Urinary System).

四、　动物实验:家兔脂肪栓塞 Animal experiment: fat embolism in rabbits

取家兔一只,自耳缘静脉注射食用植物油5~8 mL,观察兔的反应。待兔子死亡后解剖胸腔,观察其肺、心情况,然后取其部分肺脏做冰冻切片及苏丹Ⅲ染色,置于显微镜下观察,可见有多量橘红色脂肪小滴栓塞于肺泡壁毛细血管内。

请讨论兔的死亡原因。

One rabbit is injected with edible vegetable oil 5 − 8 mL from ear margin vein to observe the rabbit's reaction. After the death of the rabbit, the thoracic cavity is dissected, and the lungs and hearts are observed. Some of the lungs were frozen and stained with Sudan Ⅲ. After observation under the microscope, many orange fat droplets are embolized in alveolar wall capillaries.

Please discuss the cause of the rabbit's death.

五、　病例讨论 Case discussion

（一）病例一 Case one

病例摘要：一个大面积烧伤病人在住院期间输液时曾行大隐静脉切开插管。患者后因感染性休克而死亡,死后尸检发现髂外静脉内有血栓形成。

Case abstract：A patient with a large area of burn had undergone great saphenous vein incision and intubation during infusion during hospitalization. The patient died of septic shock. After death, thrombosis was found in the external iliac vein at autopsy.

分析题 Questions

（1）该患者血栓形成的原因是什么?

What is the cause of thrombosis in this patient?

（2）血栓是何种类型? 请描述其大体及镜下特点。

What type of thrombus is it? Describe its general and microscopic characteristics.

（二）病例二 Case two

病例摘要：女性,30 岁,自然破膜约 10 分钟后,出现寒战及呼吸困难,病情恶化,抢救无效后死亡。

尸检发现,双肺明显水肿、淤血及出血,部分区域实变,切面红褐色,多数血管内可见数量不等的有形羊水成分,如胎粪、胎脂、角化物及角化细胞等。病理诊断:双肺羊水栓塞,肺水肿。

Case abstract：A 30-year-old woman with ruptured amnion naturally died of shivering and dyspnea 10 minutes later due to deterioration of her condition.

Autopsy revealed obvious edema, congestion and hemorrhage in both lungs, consolidation in some areas, reddish-brown section, and visible amniotic fluid components in most blood vessels, such as meconium, fetal fat, keratin and keratinocytes. Pathological diagnosis was bilateral amniotic fluid embolism and pulmonary edema.

分析题 Questions

（1）羊水栓塞的发生机制是什么?

What is the mechanism of amniotic fluid embolism?

（2）试分析产妇死亡的原因。

Analyse the causes of maternal mortality.

六、 思考题 Questions

（1）何为淤血？其病理变化及后果有哪些？

What is congestion? What are the pathological changes and consequences?

（2）何为血栓形成？其形成的条件有哪些？

What is thrombosis? What are the conditions for its formation?

（3）血栓形成对机体有哪些影响？

What are the effects of thrombosis on the body?

（4）何为栓塞？栓子的运行途径有哪些？

What is embolism? What are the ways of operation of the embolus?

（5）请描述血栓栓塞的来源及其对机体的影响。

Please describe the source of thromboembolism and its effect on the body.

（6）梗死的概念是什么？梗死的类型及其形态学特点有哪些？

What is the concept of infarction? What are the types of infarction and their morphological characteristics?

编写 Written by：郭玲玲 Guo Lingling

中文审校 Chinese proofreader：邓敏 Deng Min

英文审校 English proofreader：刘瑶 Liu Yao

第四章 炎 症

Chapter 4　Inflammation

一、 教学目的 Teaching objectives

（1）掌握炎症的三种基本病理变化，了解炎症是这三种变化的综合表现。

Master the three basic pathological changes of inflammation, and understand that inflammation is a combination of these three changes.

（2）认识各种炎症细胞的形态特点及其功能。

Recognize the morphological characteristics and functions of various inflammatory cells.

（3）掌握炎症的类型及其形态特点。

Master the types of inflammation and their morphological characteristics.

二、 大体标本观察 Observation of gross specimens

（一）变质性炎 Alteration inflammation

（1）急性重型病毒性肝炎（图 4-01）：肝细胞急剧广泛坏死造成肝脏极度缩小，部分区域可见出血，在图中为黑色区域（➡）。

Acute severe viral hepatitis (Fig. 4-01): The liver is extremely reduced due to the severe necrosis of liver cells. Bleeding is visible in some areas, which are the black areas in this figure (➡).

（2）阿米巴肝脓肿（图 4-02）：在肝脏的切面上，可见直径 5 ~ 6 cm 的空腔（★），腔壁粗糙。空腔内含有灰黄色的坏死物。

Amebic liver abscess（Fig. 4-02）：On the cutting surface of the liver，there is a large cavity（5 – 6 cm in diameter）（★），the wall of which is rough. The cavity contains gray-yellow necrotic debris.

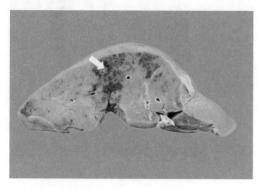

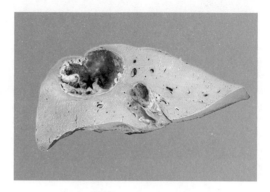

图 4-01　急性重型病毒性肝炎
Fig. 4-01　Acute severe viral hepatitis

图 4-02　阿米巴肝脓肿
Fig. 4-02　Amebic liver abscess

（二）渗出性炎 Exudation inflammation

1. 纤维素性炎 Fibrinous inflammation

（1）白喉（图 4-03）：切开的气管内有灰白色假膜（➡）被覆。

思考：咽部假膜和气管内的假膜分别对机体会引起什么样的后果？

Diphtheria（Fig. 4-03）：The cut trachea has a gray-white pseudomembrane（➡）coating.

Question：What are the consequences of the pseudomembranous membrane on the pharynx and the pseudomembrane in the trachea？

（2）纤维素性心包炎（绒毛心）（图 4-04）：脏层心包膜上覆盖着一层灰白色绒毛状纤维素（➡）。

Fibrinous pericarditis（cor hirsutum）（Fig. 4-04）：The pericardium is covered with a layer of gray-white fluffy fibrin（➡）.

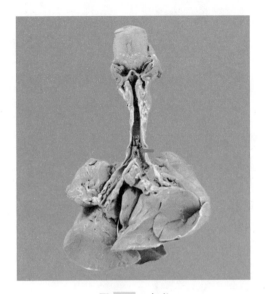

图 4-03　白喉

Fig. 4-03　Diphtheria

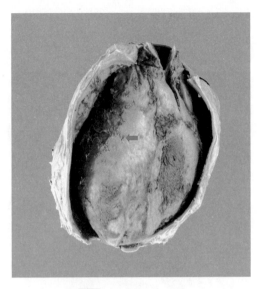

图 4-04　纤维素性心包炎

Fig. 4-04　Fibrinous pericarditis

（3）纤维素性胸膜炎（图 4-05）：胸膜明显增厚，粗糙，如破棉絮状（➡）。

Fibrinous pleuritis（Fig. 4-05）：The pleura is obviously thickened and rough, looking like the broken cotton（➡）.

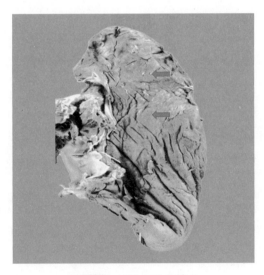

图 4-05　纤维素性胸膜炎

Fig. 4-05　Fibrinous pleuritis

2. 化脓性炎 Suppurative inflammation

（1）急性阑尾炎（图 4-06）：图中标本由上而下依次为正常阑尾、急性单纯性炎（浆膜血管明显扩张、充血）、急性蜂窝织性炎（阑尾明显肿胀、增粗，浆膜血管充血并有脓苔附着）、急性蜂窝织性炎（阑尾明显肿胀、增粗，部分颜色呈黑色）、急性坏疽性炎（阑尾大部分坏死、发黑）。

Acute appendicitis（Fig. 4-06）: Sample order from top to bottom: Normal appendix, Acute simple inflammation（the blood vessels of the serosal membrane are dilated and congested）, Acute phlegmonous inflammation（the appendix is obviously swollen and thickened, and the serosal blood vessels are congested with pus moss attached）, Acute phlegmonous inflammation（the appendix is obviously swollen and thick, and some of the color is black）, Acute gangrene inflammation（most necrosis of the appendix is black）.

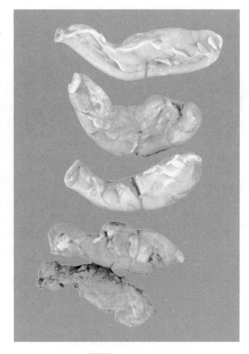

图 4-06　急性阑尾炎
Fig. 4-06　Acute appendicitis

（2）肺脓肿（图4-07）：肺切面有散在的局限性坏死灶，呈空腔状（➡），大小不一，腔内脓液已流失。

Pulmonary abscess（Fig. 4-07）: The lung section has scattered localized necrotic foci, which are hollow（➡）, of different sizes, and the pus in the cavity has lost.

（3）脑脓肿（图4-08）：大脑切面脑实质内局部组织被破坏，形成空腔（➡），空腔内脓液已经流失。

Brain abscess（Fig. 4-08）: At the brain cutting-surface, there is local tissue destruction in the brain parenchyma, forming a cavity（➡）, and the pus in the cavity has been lost.

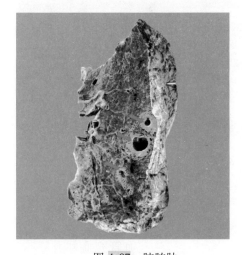

图 4-07　肺脓肿
Fig. 4-07　Pulmonary abscess

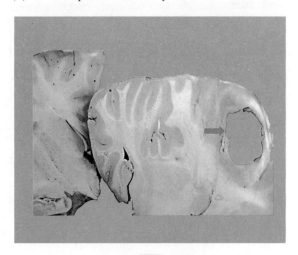

图 4-08　脑脓肿
Fig. 4-08　Brain abscess

（4）细菌性肝脓肿（图4-09）：肝切面肝实质有多个大小不等的空腔（➡），空腔内脓液已经流失。

Bacterial abscess of the liver（Fig. 4-09）：In the liver section，there are multiple cavities（➡）in the liver parenchyma，and the pus in the cavity has lost.

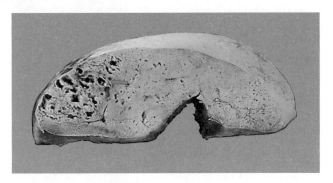

图 4-09　细菌性肝脓肿
Fig. 4-09　Bacterial abscess of the liver

（5）痈（图4-10）：皮下组织中有多个灰黄色脓肿病灶（➡），相互联通，可见有一个脓肿开口于皮肤（▲）。

Carbuncle（Fig. 4-10）：There are many gray-yellow abscess lesions（➡）in the subcutaneous tissue，which are connected to each other，and one abscess has an opening on the skin（▲）.

（6）手指窦道（图4-11）：手指末端指节肿大，表面有一窦口（➡），向下通向指骨骨髓腔。

Sinus of finger（Fig. 4-11）：The end of the finger is swollen，with a sinus opening on its surface（➡）that leads down to the medullary cavity of the phalanx.

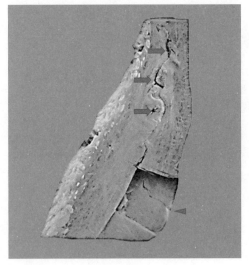

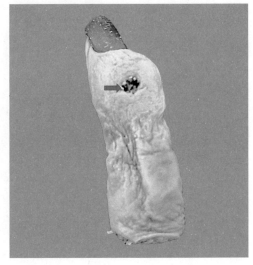

图 4-10　痈　　　　　　　　　　图 4-11　手指窦道
Fig. 4-10　Carbuncle　　　　　　Fig. 4-11　Sinus of finger

（7）肛门瘘管（图4-12）：瘘管（➡）的管壁为结缔组织。瘘管一端通向肛管（或直肠）内，另一端开口于肛门旁皮肤。

思考：窦道和瘘管有何区别？

Fistula of anus（Fig.4-12）：The wall of the fistula（➡）is connective tissue，one end of the fistula leads to the anal canal（or rectum），and the other end opens to the skin next to the anus.

Question：What are the differences between sinus and fistula？

（8）流行性脑脊髓膜炎（图4-13）：大脑表面的沟回不清，是由于灰白色脓性渗出物积聚于蛛网膜下腔所致；另外可见表面蛛网膜血管充血（➡）。

Epidemic cerebrospinal meningitis（Fig.4-13）：The sulcus on the surface of the brain is unclear due to the accumulation of grayish purulent exudate in the subarachnoid space；in addition，the surface arachnoid vessels are congested（➡）.

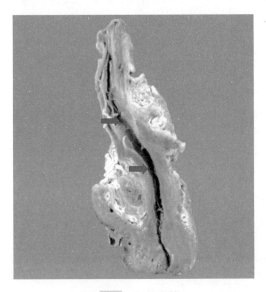

图 4-12　肛门瘘管
Fig. 4-12　Fistula of anus

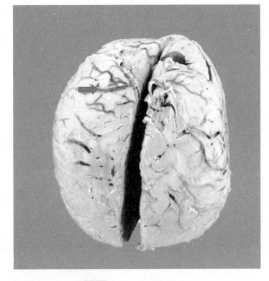

图 4-13　流行性脑脊髓膜炎
Fig. 4-13　Epidemic cerebrospinal meningitis

（三）增生性炎 Proliferation inflammation

（1）慢性扁桃体炎（图4-14）：扁桃体增大（➡），表面粗糙。

Chronic tonsillitis（Fig.4-14）：The tonsils are enlarged（➡），and the surface is rough.

（2）慢性胆囊炎、胆石症（图4-15）：胆囊壁显著增厚，有大量纤维组织增生。黏膜皱襞粗糙、扁平，丧失了正常的天鹅绒样外观。腔内有结石（➡）。

Chronic cholecystitis，cholelithiasis（Fig.4-15）：The gallbladder wall is significantly thickened，with a large amount of fibrous tissue hyperplasia. The mucosal folds are rough and flat，and the normal velvety appearance is lost. There are stones in the gallbladder cavity（➡）.

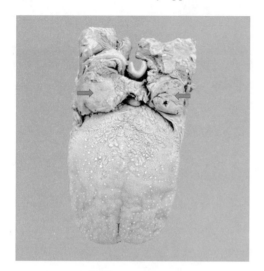

图 4-14　慢性扁桃体炎

Fig. 4-14　Chronic tonsillitis

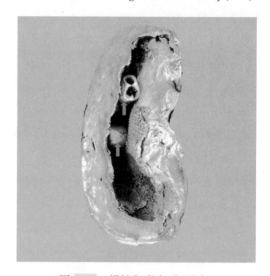

图 4-15　慢性胆囊炎、胆石症

Fig. 4-15　Chronic cholecystitis, cholelithiasis

（3）慢性血吸虫病肠炎（图 4-16）：肠壁增厚，黏膜面有许多小息肉（➡）。

Chronic schistosomiasis of the colon （Fig. 4-16）：The colonic wall is thickened and there are many small polyps （➡）on the mucosal surface.

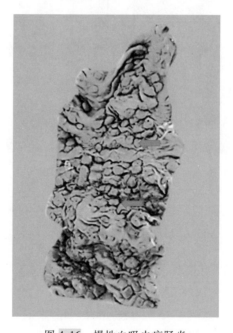

图 4-16　慢性血吸虫病肠炎

Fig. 4-16　Chronic schistosomiasis of the colon

三、组织切片观察 Observation of tissue slides

（1）扁桃体白喉（图 4-17）：扁桃体黏膜表面被覆鳞状上皮（➡）。病变处表面及隐窝内被覆一层膜状物（假膜）（▢）。假膜与其下的固有膜（▲）紧密粘连，不易脱落。假膜由网状结构的纤维素（★）和各种破碎的炎症细胞、坏死的上皮混合而成。

Tonsil diphtheria（Fig. 4-17）：The surface of the tonsil mucosa is covered with squamous epithelium（➡）. The surface of the lesion and the crypt are covered with a membrane（pseudomembrane）（▢）. The pseudomembrane closely adheres to the underlying lamina propria（▲）, which is not easy to fall off. The pseudomembrane is composed of a network of fibrin（★）and various broken inflammatory cells and necrotic epithelium.

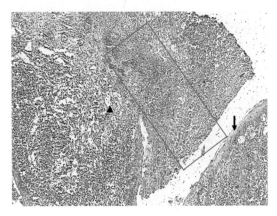
低倍镜 lower magnification

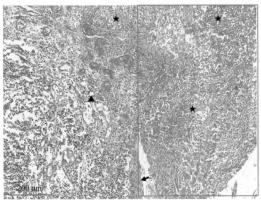
高倍镜 higher magnification

图 4-17　扁桃体白喉
Fig. 4-17　Tonsil diphtheria

（2）细菌性痢疾（图 4-18）：结肠黏膜表浅部分坏死脱落，覆盖一层膜状物（假膜）（★）；假膜由纤维素和坏死组织及炎症细胞碎屑组成，并见大量黏液（▲）；黏膜及黏膜下层充血、水肿并伴有炎症细胞浸润（➡）。

Bacterial dysentery（Fig. 4-18）：The superficial part of the colonic mucosa is necrotic and covered with a membrane（pseudomembrane）（★）. The pseudomembrane is composed of

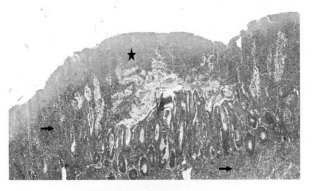
图 4-18　细菌性痢疾
Fig. 4-18　Bacterial dysentery

necrotic tissue, inflammatory cells, a large amount of mucus（▲）. Congestion, edema and inflammatory cell infiltration are found in mucosa and submucosa（➡）.

（3）急性蜂窝织性阑尾炎（图4-19）：阑尾黏膜上皮及腺体（➡）坏死（▲），阑尾腔内积脓（★）；阑尾各层的毛细血管高度扩张，充血；阑尾各层尤其是肌层（✚）明显水肿伴大量中性粒细胞弥漫浸润；中性粒细胞胞浆淡红色，胞核呈分叶状（2～5叶）（◀）。

Acute phlegmonous appendicitis（Fig.4-19）：Appendix mucosa epithelium and glands（➡）undergo necrosis（▲）. There is pus in the appendix cavity（★）. The blood vessels in appendix wall are highly dilated. In layers of the appendix, especially the muscular layer（✚）, there is obvious edema with diffuse infiltration of a large number of neutrophils; the cytoplasm of neutrophils is reddish, nucleus is lobulated（2－5 lobules）（◀）.

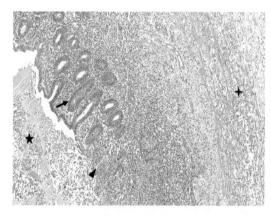

低倍镜 lower magnification　　　　　高倍镜 higher magnification

图 4-19　急性蜂窝织性阑尾炎
Fig.4-19　Acute phlegmonous appendicitis

（4）肺脓肿（图4-20）：病变部位的肺组织结构坏死消失，而代之以大量中性粒细胞局限性浸润，形成有脓液的脓腔（★）。脓液（◀）为变性坏死的中性粒细胞及坏死的组织。附近肺组织充血。肺泡内也有多少不等的浆液、纤维素（▲）及中性粒细胞。

Pulmonary abscess（Fig.4-20）：The lung tissue structure of the lesion disappears due to necrosis, and a large number of neutrophils infiltrated, forming a pus cavity（★）. The pus（◀）is

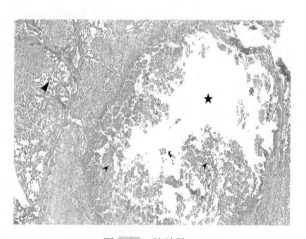

图 4-20　肺脓肿
Fig.4-20　Pulmonary abscess

composed of necrotic neutrophils and necrotic tissues. The nearby lung tissue is congested. There are also varying amounts of serum, fibrin (▲) and neutrophils in the alveoli.

（5）粟粒性肺结核病（图 4-21）：肺组织中可见散在的境界清楚的结节状病灶（✚），多数结节中央为红染、无结构、细颗粒状的干酪样坏死（▲），周围为增生的上皮样细胞（类上皮细胞）（➡）并杂有少数朗汉斯巨细胞（★）。外层有淋巴细胞（⤵）及少量纤维组织包绕。

Pulmonary military tuberculosis (Fig. 4-21): There are scattered nodular lesions with clear boundaries in the lung tissue. In the central area of most nodules, there is red-stained, unstructured, fine-grained caseous necrosis (▲), surrounded by proliferating epithelioid cells (➡) and a few Langhans' giant cells (★). There are lymphocytes (⤵) and a small amount of fibrotic tissue in the outer layer of these nodules.

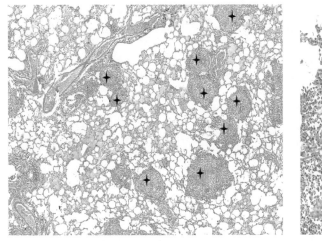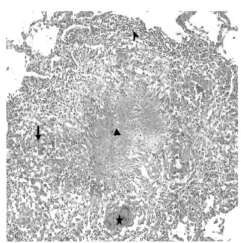

低倍镜 lower magnification   高倍镜 higher magnification

图 4-21   粟粒性肺结核病
Fig. 4-21   Pulmonary military tuberculosis

四、 病例讨论 Case discussion

（一）病例一 Case one

男性,50 岁,冬季上呼吸道感染后出现流鼻涕、流眼泪等症状。

分析题：请从病理学角度解释病人出现的临床症状。

The patient, male, 50 years old, has symptoms such as runny nose and tears in the winter due to upper respiratory tract infection.

Question: Please explain the clinical symptoms of the patient from the pathological view.

（二）病例二 Case two

男性，38 岁，颈部长疖子，伴红、肿、热、痛，10 天后局部红肿发展至手掌大，体温 38℃，局部手术切开引流，当晚即出现寒战、高热、头痛等症状。次日体检发现病人体温 39.5℃，轻度黄疸，肝脾肿大，皮肤出现瘀点，白细胞计数 21.0×10⁹/L。

分析题：请用所学的炎症知识对该病例做出病理诊断并解释上述临床表现。

The patient, male, 38 years old, got a furuncle in the neck. The furuncle is red, swollen, hot, and painful. After 10 days, the local redness and swelling lesion developed to the palm of the hand. The body temperature was 38 ℃. After the local incision and drainage surgery, symptoms, including chills, fever and headache appeared at that night. On the next day, the patient's body temperature was 39.5 ℃. Mild jaundice, hepatosplenomegaly and skin petechia were found. The WBC count was $21.0 \times 10^9/L$.

Question：Using the knowledge of inflammation, make a pathological diagnosis and explain the above clinical manifestations.

五、 思考题 Questions

（1）根据标本和切片所见，病理上如何诊断炎症？

According to the specimen and slides, how to diagnose inflammation in pathology?

（2）试述各种炎症细胞的临床意义。

Describe the clinical significance of various inflammatory cells.

（3）请叙述肉芽肿的概念及常见原因。

Please describe the concept of granuloma and its common causes.

编写 Written by：董亮 Dong Liang

中文审校 Chinese proofreader：邓敏 Deng Min

英文审校 English proofreader：刘瑶 Liu Yao

5

第五章　肿　瘤
Chapter 5　Tumors

一、　教学目的 Teaching objectives

（1）掌握肿瘤的概念及其一般形态结构。

Master the concept of tumor and its general morphological structure.

（2）掌握肿瘤的生长和扩散特点。

Master the characteristics of tumor growth and spread.

（3）掌握良恶性肿瘤以及癌与肉瘤的区别。

Master the difference between benign and malignant tumors, carcinoma and sarcoma.

（4）掌握常见肿瘤的形态及其临床特点。

Master the morphology and clinical features of common tumors.

（5）熟悉肿瘤的命名原则及分类。

Be familiar with the nomenclature and classification of tumors.

（6）熟悉肿瘤对机体的影响。

Be familiar with the effects of tumors on the body.

（7）了解肿瘤的分级与分期及病理学检查的常用方法。

Understand tumor grading and staging, and the common methods of pathological examination.

二、　大体标本观察 Observation of gross specimens

（一）肿瘤的一般特点 General characteristics of tumors

肿瘤的大体形态、数量、大小、质地、颜色及其与周围组织的关系主要与肿瘤的组织学类型、发生部位、生长方式以及良恶性性质密切相关。

The gross morphology, quantity, size, texture, color, and relationship with surrounding tissues are closely related to the histological type, location, growth pattern, and benign or malignant nature of the tumor.

1. 膨胀性生长 Expansive growth

这常常是实质器官中良性肿瘤的生长方式。肿瘤生长过程中对周围组织产生挤压,在肿瘤周围形成完整的纤维性包膜。

It is often the growth pattern of benign tumors in parenchymal organs. During the growth of the tumor, the surrounding tissue is squeezed to form a complete fibrous envelope around the tumor.

(1) 子宫平滑肌瘤(图5-01):子宫前壁已被剪开,在子宫肌层(★)可见数枚结节状的肿瘤(➡),直径0.5~4.5 cm,呈膨胀性生长,压迫周围组织形成假包膜。肿瘤与周围的子宫肌层分界清楚(➡),易于剥离。子宫内膜下也可见几枚息肉状肿瘤(▲)。

思考:内膜下的结节状肿瘤的生长方式是哪一种?

Leiomyomas of the uterine (Fig. 5-01): The anterior wall of the uterus has been cut open, and several nodular tumors (★) are seen in the myometrium (➡), ranging from 0.5 – 4.5 cm in diameter, showing expansive growth pattern. The surrounding tissue is compressed to form a pseudo-envelope, and the tumor is clearly separated from the surrounding myometrium(➡), and easy to peel off. Several polypoid tumors (▲) can also be seen under the endometrium of the uterus.

Question: What is the growth pattern of nodular tumors under the endometrium?

(2) 纤维瘤(图5-02):肿瘤表面光滑,包膜完整(★)。切面见灰白、灰黄色纵横交错的席纹状结构(➡)。

Fibroma (Fig. 5-02): The surface of the tumor is smooth and the capsule is intact (★); The cut surface is gray-white and gray-yellow, with cross stitched structures (➡).

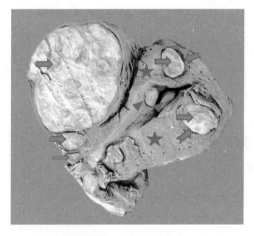

图 5-01　子宫平滑肌瘤
Fig. 5-01　Leiomyomas of the uterine

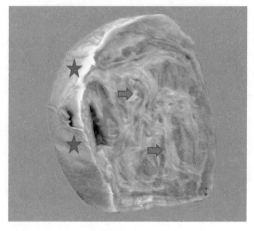

图 5-02　纤维瘤
Fig. 5-02　Fibroma

2. 外生性生长 Exogenous growth

外生性生长主要发生在体表、体腔以及有腔管道,肿瘤常突向表面,呈乳头状、息肉状、蕈伞状或菜花状。肿瘤与下方组织连接部被称为蒂部,它可以是纤长的细蒂(图 5-03),也可以呈宽蒂或没有明显的蒂部(图 5-04)。与肿瘤直接相连的组织被称为基底部。良恶性肿瘤均可呈外生性生长,但是恶性肿瘤常伴有基底部的浸润性生长(图 5-04)。

It mainly occurs in the body surface, body cavity and lumen. The tumor often protrudes to the surface, showing a papillary, polypoid, umbellate or cauliflower shape. The junction of the tumor and the underlying tissue is called the pedicle, which can be slender (Fig. 5-03), broad or without obvious pedicle (Fig. 5-04). The tissue directly connected to the tumor is called the base. Both benign and malignant tumors can be exogenous, but the malignant tumors are often accompanied by invasive growth into the basal part (Fig. 5-04).

(1) 皮肤乳头状瘤(图 5-03):肿瘤呈乳头状生长(★),有细蒂(➡)与皮肤相连(手术切除部位)。

Papilloma of the skin (Fig. 5-03): The tumor is papillary (★), with a fine pedicle (➡) attached to the skin, where could be surgically removed).

(2) 阴茎鳞状细胞癌(图 5-04):阴茎龟头部菜花状肿瘤(★),宽基底。切面可见肿瘤从基底部向下浸润,浸润至阴茎海绵体(✚),与周围组织分界不清。

Squamous cell carcinoma of the penis (Fig. 5-04): The tumor at head of the penis is cauliflower-like (★), with a broad base. The cut surface shows that the tumor infiltrates downward from the basal part, infiltrates into the corpus cavernosum (✚), and the boundary between the tumor and the surrounding tissues is not clear.

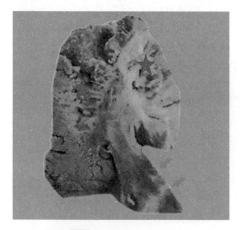

图 5-03　皮肤乳头状瘤
Fig. 5-03　Papilloma of the skin

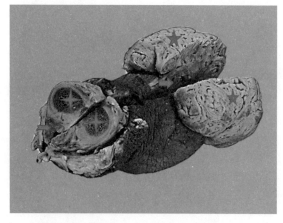

✚:正常阴茎海绵体 normal corpus cavernosum of penis;

➡:尿道海绵体 urethral corpus cavernosum.

图 5-04　阴茎鳞状细胞癌
Fig. 5-04　Squamous cell carcinoma of the penis

3. 浸润性生长 Invasive growth

肿瘤组织长入周围组织,肿瘤与周围组织境界不清(图 5-05、图 5-06),这常常是恶性肿瘤的生长方式。

Tumor tissues grow into surrounding tissues, and the boundary between tumors and surrounding tissues is not clear (Fig. 5-05 and Fig. 5-06), which is often the growth mode of malignant tumors.

（1）乳腺癌（图5-05）：乳房切面的脂肪组织内,肿瘤呈灰白色(★),无包膜。肿瘤组织向周围脂肪内呈蟹足状(树根状)浸润性生长(➡)。乳头内陷(➡),胸大肌未见明显浸润。

Breast carcinoma (Fig. 5-05): In the adipose tissue of the breast section, the tumor is grayish white (★), without a capsule. The tumor tissue is crab-like (tree root-like), invading in the surrounding fat (➡). Nipple depression (➡) could be found, and there is no significant infiltration into the pectoralis major muscle.

（2）胃癌（图5-06）:这是一个部分胃切除标本,胃壁已被剖开,局部正常的胃黏膜皱襞(▲)消失。灰白色肿瘤位于幽门管处(★),弥漫浸润到胃壁肌层(➡)。肿瘤与周围组织之间无包膜。

Gastric carcinoma (Fig. 5-06): This is a partial gastrectomy specimen, the stomach wall has been dissected, and the local normal gastric mucosal folds (▲) disappear. The gray-white tumor is located at the pyloric canal (★), diffusely infiltrating into the muscular layer of the stomach wall (➡). There is no envelope between the tumor and the surrounding tissue.

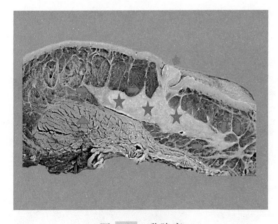

图 5-05 乳腺癌
Fig. 5-05 Breast carcinoma

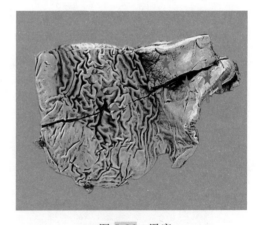

图 5-06 胃癌
Fig. 5-06 Gastric carcinoma

（二）肿瘤的转移 Metastasis of tumors

肿瘤最重要的生物学行为是转移。肿瘤的浸润性生长是肿瘤转移的前提条件。常见的肿瘤转移途径如下:

The most important biological behavior of tumors is metastasis. The invasive growth of tumors is the prerequisite for metastasis. The common ways of metastasis are as follows:

1. 淋巴道转移 Lymphatic metastasis

（1）胃癌伴淋巴结转移（图5-07）：胃窦部见不规则浸润性肿块（★）。肿块浸润到肌层。浆膜胃小弯侧淋巴结肿大（➡），有癌转移。

Carcinoma of the stomach with metastasis of the lymph node（Fig. 5-07）：An irregular infiltrative mass is seen in the antrum of the stomach（★）. The mass infiltrates into the muscle layer. Lymph nodes at the serosal small curve of the stomach（➡）, see cancer metastasis.

（2）阴茎癌伴淋巴结转移（图5-08）：阴茎龟头部菜花状肿瘤呈浸润性生长（★），另见腹股沟淋巴结转移（➡）（手术切除标本）。

Carcinoma of the penis with metastasis of the lymph node（Fig. 5-08）：The cauliflower-like tumors in the head of the penile turtle grow invasively（★）. See also the inguinal lymph node metastasis（➡）（surgical resected specimens）.

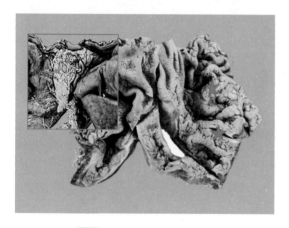

图 5-07　胃癌伴淋巴结转移
Fig. 5-07　Carcinoma of the stomach with metastasis of the lymph node

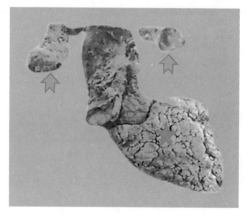

图 5-08　阴茎癌伴淋巴结转移
Fig. 5-08　Cancer of the penis with metastasis of the lymph node

（3）肺癌伴肺门淋巴结转移（图5-09）：一侧肺组织中可见弥漫的灰白色肿瘤组织（★）（弥漫性肺癌），隆突下淋巴结及肺门淋巴结均可见灰白色转移灶（➡）。

Lung cancer with hilar lymph node metastasis（Fig. 5-09）：Diffuse gray-white tumor tissue（diffuse lung cancer）can be seen in one side of the lung tissue, and grayish white metastasis are seen in subcarinal lymph nodes and hilar lymph nodes.

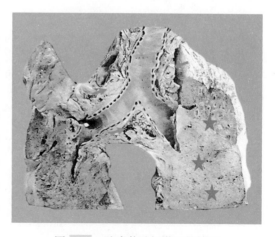

图 5-09　肺癌伴肺门淋巴结转移
Fig. 5-09　Lung cancer with hilar lymph node metastasis

2. 血道转移 Hematogenous metastasis

（1）肝转移性恶性肿瘤（图5-10）：肝切面上可见大小不等的结节状肿瘤（★），靠近肝脏表面，境界比较清楚，但无包膜。肿瘤呈棕褐色，伴有明显坏死，部分病灶伴有出血（➡）（固定后呈灰黑色）。

Metastatic malignant tumor of the liver（Fig. 5-10）：Nodular tumors（★）of various sizes can be seen on the liver section, close to

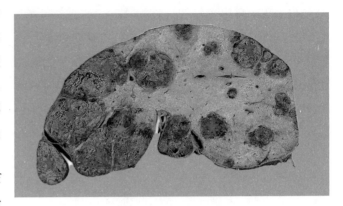

图 5-10 肝转移性恶性肿瘤

Fig. 5-10 Metastatic malignant tumor of the liver

the liver surface, and the boundary is clear, but no capsule. The tumors are brown with obvious necrosis, and some lesions are accompanied by hemorrhage（➡）（grey-black after fixation）.

（2）脑转移性恶性肿瘤（图5-11）：脑切面可见数枚境界清楚的结节状病灶（➡），无包膜。这些是脑部转移肿瘤病灶。

Metastatic malignant tumor of the brain（Fig. 5-11）：On the section of the brain, several well-defined nodular lesions（➡）（without capsule）are seen, which are metastatic lesions of the brain.

（3）脾转移性癌（图5-12）：切面见两枚直径1~2 cm、境界清楚的灰白色结节（➡），无包膜。结节经组织学证实为肿瘤转移灶。

Metastatic carcinoma of the spleen（Fig. 5-12）：Two gray-white nodules（➡）（1~2 cm in diameter）with clear boundary（without capsule）are seen on the section. Histologically, they are proved to be metastatic foci.

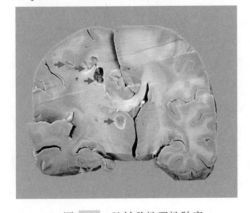

图 5-11 脑转移性恶性肿瘤

Fig. 5-11 Metastatic malignant tumor of the brain

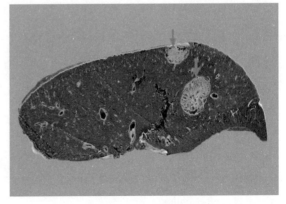

图 5-12 脾转移性癌

Fig. 5-12 Metastatic carcinoma of the spleen

3. 种植性转移 Implantable metastasis

种植性转移(图5-13):一块横膈组织(➡),表面可见大小不一的灰褐色结节状或乳头状病灶(★)。这些是肿瘤种植性转移所致。

Implantable metastasis (Fig. 5-13): On the surface of a piece of diaphragm (➡), there are taupe nodular or papillary lesions with various sizes (★). These are caused by tumor metastasis.

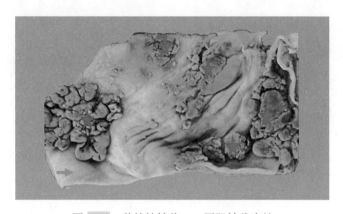

图 5-13　种植性转移——膈肌转移病灶
Fig. 5-13　Implantable metastasis—diaphragmatic metastasis

(三) 常见肿瘤 Common tumors

1. 良性上皮组织肿瘤 Benign epithelial tissue tumors

所有良性上皮性肿瘤的命名,均为组织名称后加上"瘤"字,还可以加上形态学的描写。

All benign epithelial tumors are named after the tissue name with "tumors", and the morphological description can also be added.

(1) 皮肤乳头状瘤:见图5-03。

Papilloma of the skin: See Figure 5-03.

(2) 大肠息肉样腺瘤(图5-14):肿瘤呈息肉状(★),自黏膜面(➡)向肠腔内突出生长,有蒂(➡)与肠黏膜相连,并可见局灶肠套叠(▲)。

Polypoid adenoma of the colon (Fig. 5-14): The tumor is polypoid (★) from the mucosal surface (➡) to the intestine cavity, and the pedicle(➡) is attached to the intestinal mucosa, and the focal intussusception is seen (▲).

(3) 家族性腺瘤性息肉病(图5-15):切开的一段肠管,黏膜正常皱襞消失,被无数个带蒂的息肉状肿瘤取代。此病伴有遗传学基因改变,癌变率很高。

Familial adenomatous polyposis (Fig. 5-15): A segment of the intestine was cut. The normal fold of the mucosa disappeared, and was replaced by numerous pedicled polypoid tumors.

The disease was accompanied by genetic alterations, with a high risk to be malignant.

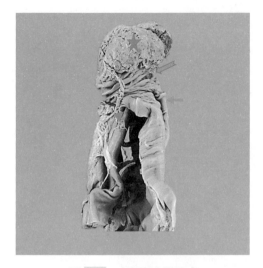

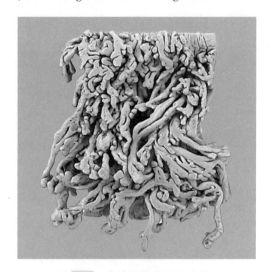

图 5-14　大肠息肉样腺瘤

Fig. 5-14　Polypoid adenoma of the colon

图 5-15　家族性腺瘤性息肉病

Fig. 5-15　Familial adenomatous polyposis

（4）卵巢黏液性囊腺瘤（图 5-16）：卵巢正常结构完全消失，被巨大的囊性肿瘤取代。肿瘤表面光滑（➡），切面为多囊性（★），囊壁较薄而光滑（➡），内含黏液（▲）。

Ovarian mucinous cystadenoma (Fig. 5-16): The normal structure of the ovary disappears completely, and is replaced by a huge cystic tumor. The surface of the tumor is smooth (➡), the cut surface is polycystic (★), and the wall of the capsule is thin and smooth (➡), containing mucus (▲).

（5）卵巢浆液性囊腺瘤（图 5-17）：已被切开的单囊性肿瘤，局灶可见残留的卵巢组织（★）。囊内容物已经流失，囊壁薄，囊内壁光滑（➡）。

Ovarian serous cystadenoma (Fig. 5-17): A single cystic tumor has been dissected, and the residual ovarian tissue(★) is found focally. The contents of the capsule have been lost, the wall of the capsule is thin, and the inner wall of the capsule is smooth (➡).

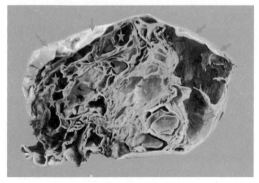

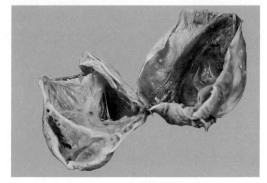

图 5-16　卵巢黏液性囊腺瘤

Fig. 5-16　Ovarian mucinous cystadenoma

图 5-17　卵巢浆液性囊腺瘤

Fig. 5-17　Ovarian serous cystadenoma

（6）多形性腺瘤（图5-18）：属于唾液腺肿瘤。肿瘤表面包膜完整（➡），切面可见透明及灰白致密条索状成分混杂（★）。

Pleomorphic adenoma（Fig. 5-18）：It belongs to the salivary gland tumor. The tumor surface envelope is intact（➡）, and the cut surface can be seen as a mixture of transparent and gray-white dense strip-like components（★）.

2. 恶性上皮性肿瘤 Malignant epithelial tumors

恶性上皮性肿瘤的命名为组织起源名称后面加上"癌"字，也可以加上形态学描述。请注意恶性肿瘤的生长方式和大体形态特点。

The malignant epithelial tumors are named after the origin of the tissue plus "carcinoma". Morphological description can also be added.

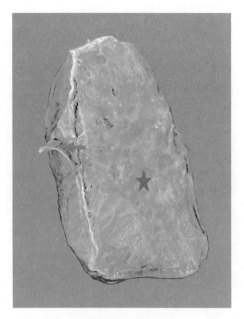

图 5-18　多形性腺瘤
Fig. 5-18　Pleomorphic adenoma

Please pay attention to the growth mode and general morphological characteristics of malignant tumors.

（1）鳞状细胞癌（squamous cell carcinoma）：鳞状细胞癌发生于鳞状上皮被覆的部位，或发生了鳞状上皮化生的地方，如肺癌。肿瘤常呈结节状、菜花状等，形态不一。多数肿瘤呈灰白色、干燥的外观，表面可形成深浅程度不一的溃疡面等，切面常可见明显的浸润性生长。

Squamous cell carcinoma：It occurs in areas covered by squamous epithelium or in areas that underwent squamous metaplasia, such as lung cancer. Tumors are often nodular, cauliflower-like, or with different forms. Most tumors have a gray-white dry appearance, and the surface can form an ulcer surface with varying degrees of defects, and the cut surface is usually infiltrated.

① 手部皮肤鳞状细胞癌（图5-19）：肿瘤位于手部皮肤。肿瘤（★）在皮肤表面外生性生长，没有蒂。肿瘤基底部比较固定，并向周围皮肤浸润（➡）；肿瘤表面有糜烂和局部出血。

Squamous cell carcinoma of the hand skin（Fig. 5-19）：The tumors are located in the hand skin. Tumors（★）grow exogenously from the skin surface without pedicles. The base of the tumors is relatively fixed and infiltrates into the surrounding skin（➡）. There is erosion and local bleeding on the surface of the tumors.

② 阴茎鳞状细胞癌（图 5-20）：阴茎龟头部肿瘤外生性生长（★）伴有浸润，肿瘤已经浸润到阴茎海绵体（➡），肿瘤与周围组织分界不清。

Squamous cell carcinoma of the penis（Fig. 5-20）：Tumor of the head of penile grew exogenously（★）accompanied by infiltration. Tumor has infiltrated into the corpus cavernosum（➡）, and the demarcation between the tumor and surrounding tissues is not clear.

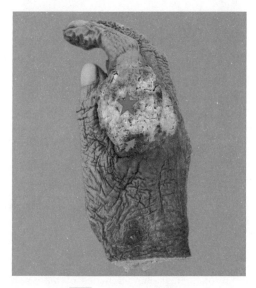
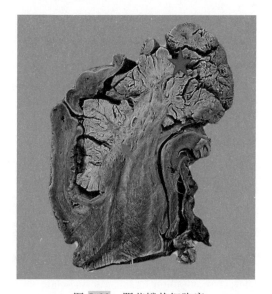

图 5-19　手部皮肤鳞状细胞癌

Fig. 5-19　Squamous cell carcinoma of the hand skin

图 5-20　阴茎鳞状细胞癌

Fig. 5-20　Squamous cell carcinoma of the penis

③ 喉鳞状细胞癌（图 5-21）：切开的喉室局部可见外生性肿瘤（★），同时肿瘤浸润至甲状软骨（➡）。

Laryngeal squamous cell carcinoma（Fig. 5-21）：An exogenous neoplasm（★）was seen locally in the incised laryngeal chamber and the tumor infiltrated into thyroid cartilage（➡）.

④ 食管鳞癌（图 5-22）：切开的一段食管中央可见不规则且边缘明显隆起（➡）的溃疡型肿块（★），肿瘤浸润到肌层甚至食管全层（➡）。

Esophageal squamous cell carcinoma（Fig. 5-22）：In the center of the esophagus that is cut, an ulcer-like mass（★）with irregular and sharp edges（➡）is seen. The tumor infiltrates into the muscular layer and even the full layer of esophagus（➡）.

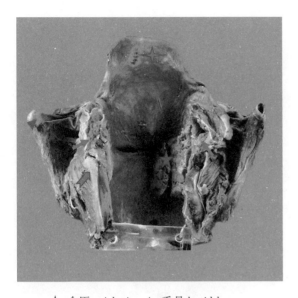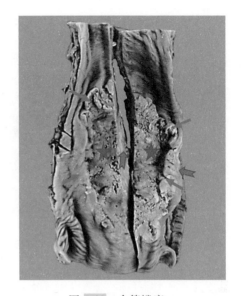

＋:会厌 epiglottis；▲:舌骨 hyoid bone；

➡:甲状软骨 thyroid cartilage.

图 5-21 喉鳞状细胞癌

Fig. 5-21 Laryngeal squamous cell carcinoma

图 5-22 食管鳞癌

Fig. 5-22 Esophageal squamous cell carcinoma

（2）腺癌：腺癌为腺上皮起源的恶性肿瘤,多见于胃肠道、肺、乳腺和女性生殖系统。不同部位的肿瘤形态不一。

Adenocarcinoma：Adenocarcinoma is a malignant tumor of glandular epithelium origin, which is more common in the gastrointestinal tract, lung, breast and female reproductive system. The tumors in different parts show different forms.

① 大肠腺癌(图 5-23)：肿瘤呈息肉状或溃疡状,或呈环状,突向肠腔或围绕肠壁生长,肠壁被浸润破坏。本例是外生性生长伴浸润性肿瘤。请自己描述肿瘤的特点。

Colorectal adenocarcinoma（Fig. 5-23）：The tumor could be polypoid, ulcerative, or annular, protruding into or surrounding the intestinal wall, and the intestinal wall is invaded and destroyed. This case is an exogenous growth with invasive tumor. Please describe the characteristics of the tumors yourself.

② 胃腺癌(图 5-24)：肿瘤的形态类型很多,本例是溃疡型肿瘤。请自己描述肿瘤的形态特点,注意癌性溃疡的特点。

Gastric adenocarcinoma（Fig. 5-24）：There are many morphological types of tumors. This case is ulcer-type tumors. Please describe the morphological characteristics of tumors and pay attention to the characteristics of cancerous ulcers.

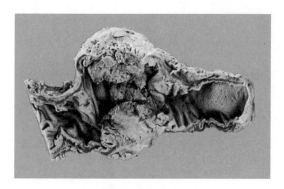

图 5-23　大肠腺癌

Fig. 5-23　Colorectal adenocarcinoma

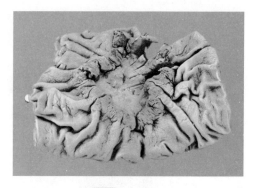

图 5-24　胃腺癌

Fig. 5-24　Gastric adenocarcinoma

③ 子宫内膜腺癌（图 5-25）：子宫前壁已被剖开，子宫腔内充满了灰白色肿瘤（★），局部明显浸润子宫肌层（➡）。

Endometrial adenocarcinoma（Figure 5-25）：The anterior wall of the uterus has been dissected, and the uterine cavity is filled with gray-white tumors（★）, with obvious local infiltration into the myometrium（➡）.

④ 乳腺癌：见图 5-05。

Breast cancer：See Fig. 5-05.

（3）尿路上皮癌：是一种起源于膀胱及肾盂被覆尿路上皮的恶性肿瘤。

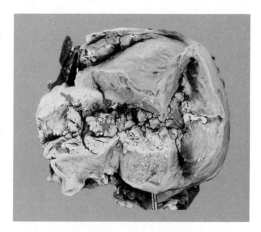

图 5-25　子宫内膜腺癌

Fig. 5-25　Endometrial adenocarcinoma

Urothelial carcinoma：A malignant tumor originating from the bladder and renal pelvis covering the urothelium.

① 膀胱尿路上皮乳头状癌（图 5-26）：膀胱已被剖开，散在以外生性生长为主的灰白色肿瘤（★）局部浸润膀胱壁（➡）。

Urothelial papillary carcinoma of bladder（Fig. 5-26）：The bladder has been dissected, and the gray-white tumor（★）, mainly exogenous growth, is partially infiltrated into the bladder wall（➡）.

② 肾盂尿路上皮乳头状癌（图 5-27）：癌组织起自肾盂（➡）黏膜并呈菜花状或乳头状生长（★），大部分肾盂为癌所充填，癌组织还向肾实质内浸润生长（➡）。

Urothelial papillary carcinoma of the renal pelvis（Fig. 5-27）：The tumors originate from the pelvic mucosa（➡）and grow in the cauliflower or papillary shape（★）. Most of the pelvis is filled by the tumors, and the cancer tissue also infiltrates into the renal parenchyma（➡）.

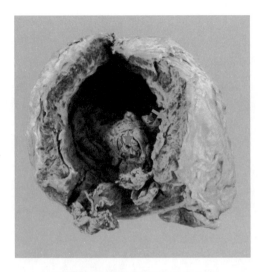

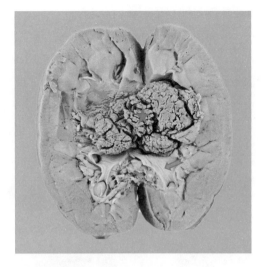

图 5-26　膀胱尿路上皮乳头状癌　　　　　图 5-27　肾盂尿路上皮乳头状癌

Fig. 5-26　Urothelial papillary carcinoma of bladder　　Fig. 5-27　Urothelial papillary carcinoma
of the renal pelvis

3. 良性间叶组织肿瘤 Benign mesenchymal tumors

间叶组织的类型很多,发生的肿瘤也比较多。良性肿瘤的命名为组织起源名称后加上
"瘤"字。常见的良性间叶组织肿瘤类型是脂肪瘤、平滑肌瘤与血管瘤。

There are many types of mesenchymal tissue, and there are many tumor types. The benign
tumors are named after the origin of the tissue plus "-oma". The common types are lipoma,
leiomyoma and hemangioma.

（1）脂肪瘤:为最常见的良性间叶组织肿瘤,多见于体表皮下组织。本例发生在肠
壁,肿瘤从肠壁黏膜面向肠腔呈外生性生长(图 5-28)。肿瘤包膜完整,表面与切面均呈黄
色(★),肿瘤引起的梗阻导致肠腔(➡)明显扩张。

思考:该肿瘤对机体的影响是什么?

Lipoma: It is the most common benign mesenchymal tissue tumor, which often occurs in the
subcutaneous tissue. This case occurs in the intestinal wall, and the tumor grows exogenously
from the mucosa of the intestinal wall to the intestinal lumen(Fig. 5-28). The tumor capsule is
intact. The surface and the cut surface are both yellow (★), and the intestinal lumen is
significantly dialated due the lipoma's obstruction (➡).

Question: What is the impact of the tumor on the body?

（2）子宫平滑肌瘤:见图 5-01。

Uterine leiomyoma: See Fig. 5-01.

（3）肝海绵状血管瘤(图 5-29):这是一个肝部分切除标本。切面可见散在多灶性的
海绵状血管腔隙病变(➡),中间或边缘杂有少量肝组织(★)。肿瘤组织无包膜。肿瘤在

肝组织中呈明显的浸润性生长。

Spongyhemangioma of the liver（Fig. 5-29）：This is a partially resected specimens of the liver. Multifocal spongy vascular cavity lesions（➡）could be seen in the cut surface, with a small amount of liver tissue（★）in the middle or at the edge. The tumor has no envelope. The tumor grows invasively in the liver tissue.

（4）纤维瘤（fibroma）：见图5-02。

Fibroma：See Fig. 5-02.

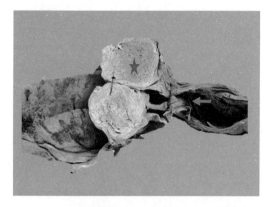 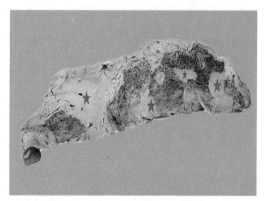

图 5-28　肠壁脂肪瘤　　　　　　　　　图 5-29　肝海绵状血管瘤

Fig. 5-28　Intestinal lipoma　　　　　　Fig. 5-29　Spongyhemangioma of the liver

4. 恶性间叶组织肿瘤 Malignant mesenchymal tissue tumors

间叶组织起源的恶性肿瘤被称为肉瘤。肉瘤占恶性肿瘤的比例较小，但是类型却比较复杂，诊断比较困难。

Malignant tumors originating from mesenchymal tissue are called sarcomas, which accounts for a small proportion of malignant tumors, but its types are complex and difficult to diagnose.

（1）骨肉瘤（图5-30）：肿瘤位于股骨下端。灰白色肿瘤组织从骨髓腔发生（★），破坏骨皮质并穿透骨膜（➡），侵及软组织（▲）。切面病变处呈梭形肿胀，骨膜被瘤组织顶起（➡），骨皮质与掀起的骨膜形成X线上的 Codmas 三角。

Osteosarcoma（Fig. 5-30）：The tumor is located at the lower end of the femur. Grayish white tumor tissue develops from the medullary cavity（★）, breaks the cortical bone, penetrates the periosteum（➡）, and invades the soft tissue（▲）. The cut surface shows spindle-shaped swelling, the periosteum is uplifted by the tumor tissue（➡）, and the cortical bone and the sclered periosteum forms the Codmas triangle on the X-ray.

（2）软骨肉瘤（图5-31）：胫骨平台肿瘤呈灰白色，半透明（➡），略呈分叶状，从骨髓腔侵犯周围软组织（★）。

Chondrosarcoma（Fig. 5-31）：The tumor of the tibial plateau is gray and semi-translucent

（ ➡ ），slightly lobulated，and invading the surrounding soft tissue from the bone marrow cavity（ ★ ）.

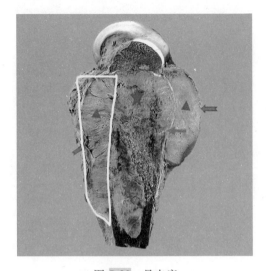

图 5-30　骨肉瘤

Fig. 5-30　Osteosarcoma

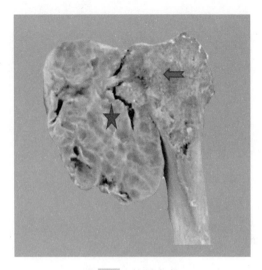

图 5-31　软骨肉瘤

Fig. 5-31　Chondrosarcoma

（3）血管肉瘤：皮肤中央可见灰黑色(新鲜标本常呈暗红色)隆起肿块,呈浸润性生长（图 5-32）。

Angiosarcoma：There is a gray and black（dark red in fresh specimen）bulging mass in the center of the skin，growing invasively（Fig. 5-32）.

（4）纤维肉瘤（图 5-33）：儿童患者一侧前臂可见肿瘤。肿瘤自肘关节附近皮下组织弥漫向周围浸润生长,形成巨大肿块。肿瘤浸润性生长,与周围组织之间界限不清;切面呈灰白色略带粉红色,质地均匀,杂有交错的纤维索状结构,已侵犯骨组织。

Fibrosarcoma（Fig. 5-33）：There is a tumor in one side of the forearm from a child patient. The tumor grows from the subcutaneous tissue near the elbow and invades diffusely into the surrounding tissues，forming a huge mass. The tumor grows invasively，with unclear boundary from the surrounding tissues；the cut surface is grayish white with a slight pink color，uniform texture，and intertwined fiber-like structure，which has invaded the bone tissue.

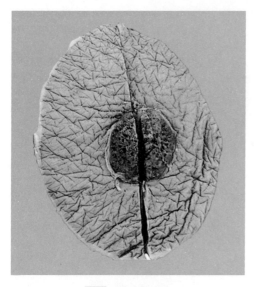

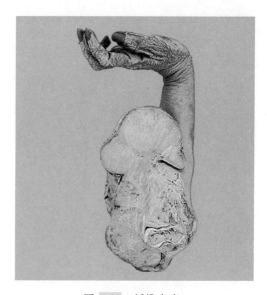

图 5-32　皮肤血管肉瘤

Fig. 5-32　Angiosarcoma of the skin

图 5-33　纤维肉瘤

Fig. 5-33　Fibrosarcoma

5. 神经外胚叶肿瘤 Neuroectodermal tumors

（1）小脑星形细胞瘤（图 5-34）：脑组织正中矢状切面可见小脑半球肿大（★）。肿瘤呈囊性变（➡），囊壁光滑,囊壁可见附壁结节（➡）。

Cerebellar astrocytoma（Fig. 5-34）：On the mid-sagittal section of brain tissue, there is enlargement of cerebellar hemisphere（★）. There is cystic change（➡）in the tumor, with smooth cystic wall and mural nodule（➡）.

（2）脑膜瘤（图 5-35）：该标本为手术完整剥离的肿瘤。肿瘤呈球形,有完整包膜（★）。瘤组织致密、灰白,部分有明显细条索状物（▲）。

Meningioma（Fig. 5-35）：This specimen is a tumor after a complete surgical dissection. The tumor is spherical, with a complete capsule（★）. The tumor tissue is dense, grayish, and some area sees obvious thin cords（▲）.

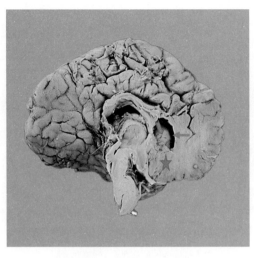

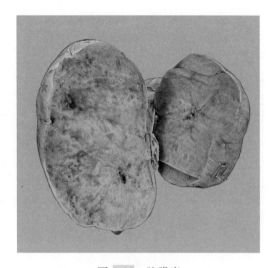

图 5-34　小脑星形细胞瘤　　　　　　　图 5-35　脑膜瘤
Fig. 5-34　Cerebellar astrocytoma　　　Fig. 5-35　Meningioma

（3）黑色素瘤：肿瘤位于足趾部（图 5-36），表面有溃疡形成。肿瘤表面及切面均呈深褐色或黑色（➡）。瘤组织向周围浸润生长，趾骨已被破坏（★）。

Melanoma：The tumor is located on the toe（Fig. 5-36），with ulceration in its surface. Its surface and the cut surface are dark brown or black（➡）. The tumor tissue infiltrates into the surrounding area and the phalanges have been destroyed（★）.

6. 其他肿瘤 Miscellaneous tumors

畸胎瘤 Teratoma

卵巢囊性成熟性畸胎瘤（图 5-37）：肿瘤为一表面光滑的囊性肿块。囊外壁即为肿瘤的包膜，切开后可见多囊性结构，囊内壁光滑（★）。囊内容物为皮脂（▲）、毛发（➡）及牙齿（➡）等。

Ovarian cystic mature teratoma（Fig. 5-37）：The tumor is a smooth cystic mass. The outer wall of the capsule is the capsule of the tumor. After incision, a polycystic structure could be seen, and the inner wall of the capsule is smooth（★）. Its content includes sebum（▲）, hair（➡）and teeth（➡）.

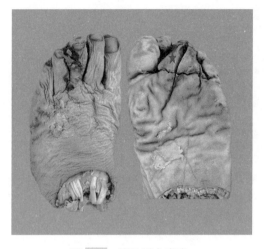

图 5-36　脚趾黑色素瘤

Fig. 5-36　Melanoma of the phalanges

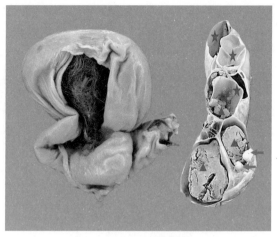

图 5-37　卵巢囊性成熟性畸胎瘤

Fig. 5-37　Ovarian cystic mature teratoma

三、　组织切片观察 Observation of tissue slides

（一）肿瘤的异型性 Atypia of neoplasms

异型性是指肿瘤组织与其起源的正常组织之间的差异,包括肿瘤的结构异型性及细胞异型性。良性肿瘤的异型性较小,主要表现为结构异型性;恶性肿瘤的异型性大,除了具有明显的组织结构异型性外,还有明显的细胞形态异型性。

Atypia is the difference between the tumor and the normal tissue from which it originates, including the architectural atypia and the cellular atypia. Benign tumors have small atypia, mainly characterized by architectural atypia, while malignant tumors have huge atypia, including obvious architectural atypia, as well as significant cellular morphological atypia.

（1）肝细胞癌（图 5-38）：与正常的肝组织（▲）相比,肝细胞癌组织（★）具有明显的异型性。

Hepatocellular carcinoma (Fig. 5-38): Compared with normal liver tissue (▲), hepatocellular carcinoma (HCC) (★) has obvious atypia.

① 结构异型性：正常肝小叶中央为中央静脉,单层排列的肝细胞板围绕中央静脉呈放射状排列,肝板之间为肝

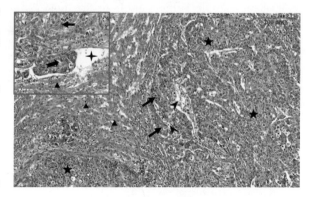

图 5-38　肝细胞癌

Fig. 5-38　Hepatocellular carcinoma

血窦;而癌组织没有可辨别的肝小叶结构,它由3~5排不等的癌细胞形成比正常肝板厚很多的肝板样结构(➡),无中央静脉,尽管肝板样结构之间可见肝窦样结构(➣)。

Architectural atypia: The central part of the normal hepatic lobules is the central vein, and the monolayer-arranged hepatocyte plates are arranged radially around the central vein, with hepatic sinus between the liver plates. While there is no discernible hepatic lobular structure in the cancer tissue. Three to five rows of cancer cells formed the liver plate-like structure, much thicker than the normal liver plate (➡). There is no central veins, although the hepatic sinusoidal structure (➣) is visible between the hepatic plate-like structures.

② 细胞异型性:正常肝细胞核小而圆,常位于肝细胞中心,核浆比为1:4~6,核分裂少见或不见。癌细胞(➡)大小不等,形态不规则,核大、深染,可见瘤巨细胞及病理学核分裂象。不同分化程度的癌细胞异型性有所不同。

Cellular atypia: Normal liver cell nucleus is small and round, and often located in the center of hepatocytes, with the ratio of nucleoplasm 1:4 − 6 and rare mitosis. While cancer cells (➡) shows different sizes, irregular shape and deep nuclear dyeing. Sometimes there is tumor giant cells and pathological mitosis. Cancer cells with different differentiation shows different degree of atypia.

③ 浸润性生长:肝细胞癌的癌细胞浸润周围正常组织(▲),脉管内(✛)可见癌栓(➡)。

Invasive growth: Hepatocellular carcinoma cells infiltrate into the surrounding normal tissues (▲), and the tumor thrombus (➡) can be seen in the vasculature (✛).

(2) 大肠绒毛状-管状腺瘤(图5-39):黏膜组织局灶增生,向肠腔呈乳头状突起部分(★)即为肿瘤,有一短蒂(▲)与肠壁相连(部分已经分离);肿瘤呈外生性生长,未见浸润。

Tubulo-villous adenoma of the colon (Fig. 5-39): The mucosal tissue is hyperplastic, and the papillary part of the intestine is a tumor. There is a short pedicle (▲) connected to the intestinal wall (partially separated); the tumor is

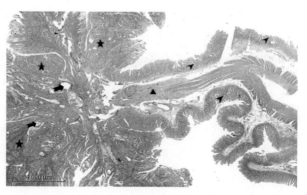

图 5-39　大肠绒毛状-管状腺瘤
Fig. 5-39　tubulo-villous adenoma of the colon

exogenously growing and no infiltration is observed.

① 结构异型性:与周围正常的大肠黏膜(➣)相比,肿瘤性腺上皮形成腺管样结构和绒毛状结构;腺腔大小不一,部分呈囊状扩张(➡),排列紊乱;绒毛状结构为腺上皮呈指状突起,其中心部分为纤维血管轴心。

Architectural atypia: Compared with the normal colorectal mucosa (✔), the tumorous glandular epithelium forms glandular duct-like structures and villous structures; the glandular cavity varies in size, partly expands cystically (➡), and is arranged disorderly. The villous structure is a finger- like protrusion of the glandular epithelium, and its center is the axis of the fibrous blood vessel.

② 细胞异型性：不明显，腺上皮细胞大小比较一致，细胞核小，基本位于细胞的基底部，核分裂少见，并可见到杯状细胞，这些与正常肠上皮细胞相似，分化成熟，提示肿瘤细胞恶性度低。

Cellular atypia: not obvious, glandular epithelial cells are relatively uniform in size, small in nucleus, located at the base of cells, and nuclear division is rare, and goblet cells can be seen, which are similar to normal intestinal epithelial cells, indicating mature differentiation, suggesting malignant low.

（3）大肠腺癌（图5-40）：正常黏膜层（黏膜肌层➡）的腺体大小一致、排列具有极性（★）。腺癌组织由大小极不一致、排列不规则的腺样结构组成（➡），亦有部分癌细胞呈索条状、片块状排列，并不形成明显的腺样结构。癌组织表面可见坏死、糜烂（✔），癌已浸润到肌层（✚）。癌细胞核大、深染，有核分裂象。

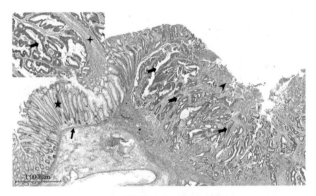

图 5-40　大肠腺癌

Fig. 5-40　Adenocarcinoma of the colon

Adenocarcinoma of the colon (Fig. 5-40): Glands in the normal mucosa (the mucosal muscle layer ➡) has the same size and polarity (★). The adenocarcinoma is composed of glands with extremely inconsistent size and irregular adenoid structure (➡), and some cancer cells are cord-like or sheet-like, without forming a distinct adenoid structure. There is necrosis and erosion at the surface of the cancer tissue (✔) and the tumor invaded into the muscular layer (✚). The cancer cell is deeply stained, with mitosis.

（二）肿瘤生长与扩散 Tumor growth and spread

（1）外生性生长——皮肤乳头状瘤、大肠绒毛状-管状腺瘤。

Exogenous growth—skin papilloma, large intestine villus-tubular adenoma.

（2）膨胀性生长——纤维瘤。

Expansive growth—fibroma.

（3）浸润性生长——大肠腺癌、皮肤鳞癌。

Invasive growth—colorectal adenocarcinoma, skin squamous cell carcinoma.

(4) 淋巴结转移性腺癌(图5-41)：淋巴结正常结构(▲为淋巴滤泡)部分被破坏，被膜下窦(◣)及边缘窦中可见条索状、片块状的癌细胞团(★)，部分癌细胞形成大小不等、形状不一、排列不规则的腺体或腺样结构。此为转移性低分化腺癌。

思考：高分化腺癌具有什么样的形态学特征？

Metastatic adenocarcinoma of the lymph node (Fig. 5-41)：The normal structure of lymph nodes (▲ is lymphoid follicle) is partially destroyed, and the subcapsular sinus (◣) and marginal sinus are seen as cord-like, patchy cancer cell mass (★), part of cancer cells form glands or adenoid structures of varying sizes, shapes, and irregularities. This is a metastatic poorly differentiated adenocarcinoma.

Question：What is the morphological feature of a highly differentiated adenocarcinoma?

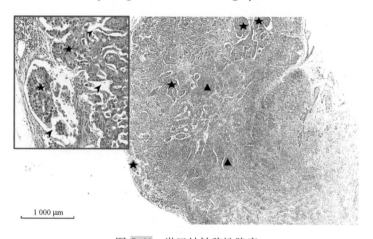

1 000 μm

图 5-41 淋巴结转移性腺癌
Fig. 5-41 Metastatic adenocarcinoma of the lymph node

(三) 良恶性肿瘤以及癌与肉瘤的区别 The difference between benign and malignant tumors, cancer and sarcoma

通过比较皮肤乳头状瘤和皮肤鳞癌、纤维瘤与纤维肉瘤，了解良性和恶性肿瘤的镜下区别；通过比较鳞癌与纤维肉瘤，了解癌与肉瘤的镜下区别。

Understand the difference between benign and malignant tumors by comparing the skin papilloma and skin squamous cell carcinoma, fibroids and fibrosarcoma under the microscope. Understand the difference between cancer and sarcoma by comparing squamous cell carcinoma with fibrosarcoma.

(1) 皮肤乳头状瘤(图5-42)：肿瘤呈乳头状外形(★)，乳头中心为纤维组织及血管，二者组成轴心(➡)，此为肿瘤的间质，其中尚可见到少量淋巴细胞及浆细胞浸润；被覆在纤维血管轴心表面的是增生的复层鳞状细胞，其底层为基底细胞(➡)，中层为增生的棘细胞层（✚），表层为颗粒细胞及明显增厚的角化层（▲），各层细胞与正常的复层鳞状上皮相似，基膜完好，无浸润现象。

Papilloma of the skin（Fig. 5-42）：Tumor is papillary shape（★）, the center of the papilla is fibrous tissue and vascular axis（➡）, which is the stroma of the tumor, in which a small amount of lymphocyte and plasma cell infiltration can be seen; the surface of the axis of the fibers and vessels is covered by proliferative stratified squamous cells, whose basal layer is basal cell（➡）, and the middle layer is proliferative spinous cells（✚）, the surface layer is granular cells and markedly thickened keratinized layer（▲）, each layer of cells is similar to a normal stratified squamous epithelium, with intact basement membrane and no infiltration.

（2）鳞状细胞癌：鳞状细胞癌是一种起源于表皮、鳞状上皮或鳞化区的恶性上皮肿瘤。

Squamous cell carcinoma is a malignant epithelial tumor which originates in epidermis, squamous mucosa or areas of squamous metaplasia.

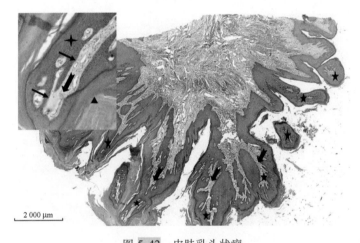

2 000 μm

图 5-42　皮肤乳头状瘤
Fig. 5-42　Papilloma of the skin

① 皮肤高分化鳞状上皮癌（图 5-43）：复层鳞状上皮高度增生并癌变。肿瘤细胞破坏基底膜，形成片状或致密块，侵入皮下结缔组织（真皮），形成大小不等的癌巢（★）。肿瘤细胞具有轻度异型性。癌巢的细胞排列方式常与正常表皮相似：边缘为未成熟的基底细胞；内层细胞类似于表皮的棘细胞（✚）（大而多角形，具有丰富的嗜酸性胞质，细胞核位于中央）；癌巢的中心为更加成熟的层状角化物，常形成同心圆排列的分层结构，称为"角化珠"（▲）；周围的间质较少，有炎细胞浸润；癌组织与周围间质（➡）分界清楚。

Well-differentiated squamous cell carcinoma of the skin（Fig. 5-43）：The stratified squamous epithelium is highly proliferative and cancerous. Tumor cells destroy the basement membrane, form lamella or dense mass, invade the subcutaneous connective tissue（dermis）, and form a nest of cancers of different sizes（★）. The tumor cells have mild atypia. The cell arrangement of the cancer nest is often similar to that of the normal epidermis. Immature basal cells locate in the nest margin, and the inner cells are similar to normal spinous cells (✛) (large and polygonal, rich in eosinophilic cytoplasm, central nucleus). The center of the nest is a more mature, layered keratin, often forming a concentric arrangement of layers, called "keratin pearl" (▲); the surrounding stroma is reduced and contains inflammatory infiltrate. The boundary between cancer tissues and the surrounding tumor stroma (➡) is clear.

② 皮肤中分化鳞状上皮癌(图5-44)：与高分化鳞癌相比,癌细胞异型性明显,细胞形态不一,核大而深染,可见大量病理性核分裂(➹),少量癌细胞间见细胞间桥(➡),少数癌细胞浆具有嗜酸性(细胞内角化),癌巢中央未见角化珠。

Moderately differentiated squamous cell carcinoma of the skin (Fig. 5-44) : Compared with highly differentiated squamous cell carcinomas, cancer cells are more atypia. Cells show different morphology, large and deep-stained nuclei and a large number of pathological mitosis (➹). A few cancer cells have intercellular bridges (➡), and a few have eosinophilic cytoplasm (intracellular keratinization), but no keratin pearl.

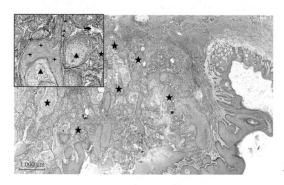

图 5-43 皮肤高分化鳞状上皮癌
Fig. 5-43 Well-differentiated squamous cell carcinoma of the skin

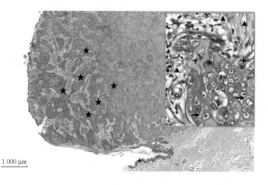

★:癌巢 nest; ➡:正常鳞状上皮 Normal squamous epithelium; ▲:肿瘤间质 tumor stroma.
图 5-44 皮肤中分化鳞状上皮癌
Fig. 5-44 Moderately differentiated squamous cell carcinoma of the skin

请注意观察皮肤乳头状瘤与皮肤鳞癌在镜下的异型性及生长方式的不同。

Pay attention to the difference in the shape and growth pattern between skin papilloma and squamous cell carcinoma under the microscope.

(3) 纤维瘤(图5-45)：瘤细胞(➡)与纤维细胞相似,细长呈梭形,核小而狭长,排列成束状、波浪状,纵横交错,无核分裂象;瘤细胞间有大量胶原纤维形成。

Fibroma (Fig. 5-45) : Tumor cells (➡) are similar to fibroblasts, slender and fusiform, with small and narrow nuclei, arranged in a bundle, wavy, and criss-cross, without mitotic figures. A large amount of collagen fibers are formed between the tumor cells.

（4）纤维肉瘤（图 5-46）：瘤细胞排列成束状、波浪状，纵横交错。与纤维瘤相比，肉瘤细胞丰富，类似成纤维细胞，呈椭圆形或梭形，胞浆少，胞核大而核膜厚，大小形态不一致，可见核分裂（ ）。局灶瘤组织坏死（ ）。与癌组织相比，肉瘤间质较少，血管丰富（ ），瘤细胞与肿瘤间质无明确界限。

Fibrosarcoma (Fig. 5-46)：Tumor cells are arranged in bundles, waves, and crisscrossed. Compared with fibroids, tumor cells are abundant, resembling fibroblasts, which are elliptical or fusiform, with less cytoplasm. The nucleus is large and the nuclear membrane is thick, the size and shape are inconsistent, and mitosis is seen（ ）. Local tumor necrosis may occur（ ）. Compared with carcinoma, there is less stroma but more vessels（ ）, and more unclear boundary between tumor cells and stroma in sarcoma.

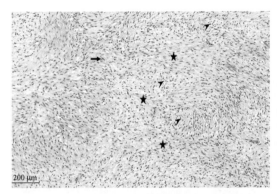

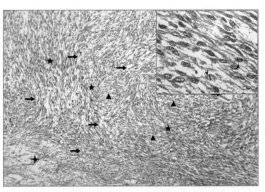

:瘤细胞的纵切面 the longitudinal section of tumor cells；★:瘤细胞的横切面 the cross-section of the tumor cells.

★:瘤细胞的纵切面 the longitudinal section of tumor cells；▲:瘤细胞的横切面 the cross-section of the tumor cells.

图 5-45　纤维瘤

Fig. 5-45　Fibroma

图 5-46　纤维肉瘤

Fig. 5-46　Fibrosarcoma

四、 病例讨论 Case discussion

宋某，男，21 岁，大学生。该学生在 3 个月前打篮球时下肢受伤后出现膝盖处间歇性隐痛，近 1 个月来病情进行性加重，膝盖下方肿胀明显伴持续性疼痛。

Song, male, 21 years old, a college student, had an intermittent pain in the knee after a knee injury during playing basketball three months ago. The pain progressively aggravated in the past month, and the swelling under the knee is obvious, accompanied by persistent pain.

体格检查:右大腿关节下方梭形肿胀伴轻度压痛。

Physical examination：Spindle swelling under the right thigh joint with tenderness.

X 线检查:右胫骨上段骨质破坏伴轻度病理性骨折。病人被收住入院后行截肢术。

X-ray examination：Upper right tibia destruction with mild pathological fracture. The patient was admitted to hospital to perform amputation.

病理检查：右胫骨上段、胫骨平台骨组织及骨髓腔大部分已被破坏,可见灰红色、鱼肉样组织。镜检可见散在针状、片状及小梁状不成熟骨样组织,骨样组织周围及小梁之间可见弥漫分布的瘤细胞,呈圆形、梭形、多边形,核大而深染,核分裂多见,间质少但血管丰富。

Pathological examination：The upper part of right tibia, tibial plateau bone tissue and the bone marrow cavity were mostly destroyed, with gray-red and fish-like tissues seen. Microscopic examination shows scattered needle-like, lamellar and trabecular immature bone-like tissues. Tumor cells around and between trabecular bone-like tissues are diffuse, round, spindle-shaped and polygonal, with large dark-stained nuclei, with common mitoses, scattered interstitial tissue and rich blood vessels.

患者被截肢后伤口愈合出院。出院后 6 个月,患者出现胸痛、咳嗽、咯血等症状,皮肤多处见肿瘤病灶。病理学检查显示组织学类似胫骨肿瘤改变,实验室检查显示血清碱性磷酸酶升高。

After amputation, the patient was discharged from hospital after wound healing. Six months after discharge, the patient developed symptoms such as chest pain, cough and hemoptysis. There are multiple tumor lesions in the skin. Pathological examination showed that the histological changes were similar to that of the tibial tumor. Laboratory examination showed elevated serum alkaline phosphatase.

分析题 Questions

（1）请根据临床及病理特点对患者右大腿肿瘤做出诊断。

Please make a diagnosis of right thigh tumor based on clinical and pathological features.

（2）请解释患者被截肢 6 个月后出现的各种临床症状。

Please explain the clinical symptoms of the patient six months after amputation.

五、 思考题 Questions

（1）请描述肿瘤性生长与非肿瘤性生长的区别。

Please describe the difference between neoplastic hyperplasia and non-neoplastic hyperplasia.

（2）举例说明肿瘤异型性的具体表现。

Give an example of the specific manifestations of tumor atypia.

（3）肿瘤有哪些生长方式？

What are the growth patterns of tumors?

（4）请描述良性肿瘤与恶性肿瘤的区别。

Please describe the difference between benign and malignant tumors.

（5）请描述癌与肉瘤的区别。

Please describe the difference between carcinoma and sarcoma.

（6）肿瘤的扩散方式有哪些？认识肿瘤扩散的基本规律有何临床意义？

What are the ways in tumors spread? What is the clinical significance of recognizing the basic law of tumor spreading?

（7）请举例说明肿瘤的命名原则。

Please give examples of the nomenclature of the tumors.

编写 Written by：邓敏 Deng Min

英文审校 English proofreader：刘瑶 Liu Yao

6

第六章　心血管系统疾病

Chapter 6　Diseases of the Heart and Blood Vessels System

一、 教学目的 Teaching objectives

（1）掌握风湿病的基本病变,熟悉慢性风湿性心瓣膜病的形态特征及其对机体的危害。

Master the pathologic change of rheumatic disease, and be familiar with the morphological characteristics of rheumatic valvular disease and their impact on the body.

（2）熟悉细菌性心内膜炎的形态特征及临床联系。

Be familiar with the morphological characteristics and clinical features of infective endocarditis.

（3）掌握高血压病的病变特点及其对机体的危害。

Master the morphological characteristics of hypertension and their impact on the body.

（4）掌握动脉粥样硬化症的主要病变特点及其对机体的危害。

Master the morphological characteristics of atherosclerosis and their impact on the body.

二、 大体标本观察 Observation of gross specimens

（一）正常心脏 Normal heart

正常心脏(图6-01):成人心脏大小与本人左拳相似,重250 g左右,左室壁厚1 cm(★),右室壁厚0.3～0.4 cm,心房壁厚0.2 cm;心瓣膜(➡)及心内膜光滑、菲薄、透明,各瓣膜附着缘不粘连,腱索细而光滑,乳头肌亦不肥大。各瓣膜口周径如下:三尖瓣11 cm,肺动脉瓣8.5 cm,二尖瓣10 cm,主动脉瓣7.5 cm。

Normal heart (Fig. 6-01): The size of an adult's heart is the same as his left fist. And the weight of heart is about 250 g. The left ventricle normally has a wall thickness of up to 1 cm (★) , the wall of right ventricle is about 0. 3 – 0. 4 cm, and the wall of atrium is 0. 2 cm. The valves (➡) and pericardium are smooth, thin and transparent. The attachment edges of the valves are not adhered, the tendons are thin and smooth, and the papillary muscles are not hypertrophied. The circumference of each valve is as follows：The diameter of tricuspid valve, pulmonary valve, mitral valve and aortic valve are 11 cm, 8. 5 cm, 10 cm, and 7. 5 cm respectively.

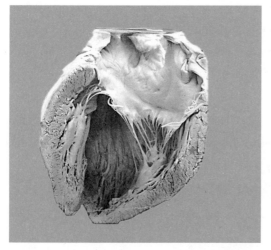
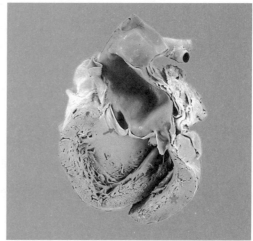

图 6-01　正常心脏

Fig. 6-01　Normal heart

（二）动脉粥样硬化症 Atherosclerosis

（1）主动脉粥样硬化（图6-02）：主动脉内膜粗糙不平,有扁平且略隆起的呈圆形或不规则的斑块(➡),淡黄色或灰白色,有的形成粥样溃疡或有钙化(★)。

Atherosclerosis of the aorta（Fig. 6-02）：The aortic intima is rough and flat, with a slightly rounded or irregular plaque （ ➡ ）. The surface shows canary yellow or grey atherosclerotic plaques. Some of plaques associated with ulceration or calcification(★).

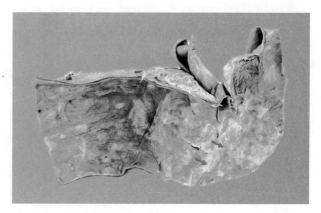

图 6-02　主动脉粥样硬化

Fig. 6-02　Atherosclerosis of the aorta

（2）心肌梗死（图6-03）：左心室前壁心尖部分心肌结构不清、变薄,组织疏松并失去光泽(➡),心室内壁可见附壁血栓形成(★)。

Myocardial infarction (Fig. 6-03)：The infracted zone, which is pale, thin and lost normal structure, includes the anterior of left ventricle(➡), and anterior myocardial infarct with mural thrombus(★).

（3）脑动脉粥样硬化(图 6-04)：脑基底动脉环(Willis 环)及其分支节段性硬化,呈竹节状,硬化区可见黄色或灰黄色斑块(➡)。

Atherosclerosis of the cerebral arteries (Fig. 6-04)：The surface of the Willis Circle and its branches shows sclerosis, which is similar to bamboo. The sclerotic area are yellow or grey yellow atherosclerotic plaques(➡).

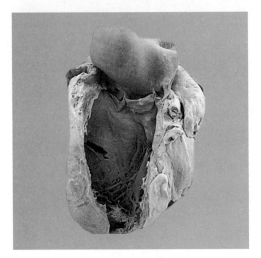

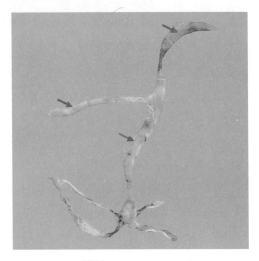

图 6-03　心肌梗死

Fig. 6-03　Myocardial infarction

图 6-04　脑动脉粥样硬化

Fig. 6-04　Atherosclerosis of the cerebral arteries

（4）肾动脉粥样硬化(图 6-05)：肾脏体积缩小,表面可见楔形梗死区,已疤痕化(➡)。

Atherosclerosis of the renal arteries (Fig. 6-05)：The size of the kidney was reduced, and wedge-shaped infarct area was seen on the surface, and the infracted zone was scarred(➡).

（三）高血压病 Hypertension

（1）高血压心脏病(图6-06)：左心室肥厚(★)(正常厚度为0.8~1 cm),乳头肌及肉柱均增粗。有些标本的左心室已明显扩张。

思考:左心室扩张说明了什么?

Hypertensive cardiopathy (Fig. 6-06)：Left ventricular becomes hypertrophic (normal thickness 0.8 – 1 cm), papillary muscle and meat column are enlarged, and some left ventricular wall is apparently thickened(★).

Question：What does the left ventricular enlargement indicate?

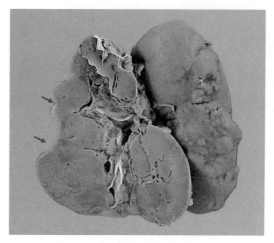

图 6-05　肾动脉粥样硬化

Fig. 6-05　Atherosclerosis of the renal arteries

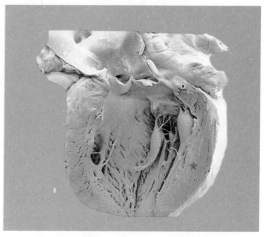

图 6-06　高血压心脏病

Fig. 6-06　Hypertensive cardiopathy

（2）高血压肾病（图 6-07）（原发性颗粒固缩肾）：肾体积缩小，表面不平，呈细颗粒状
（➡）。

Hypertensive kidney（Fig. 6-07）（Primary granular atrophy of the kidney）：The kidney with small, progressive fibrosis and granular appearance（➡）.

（3）高血压脑出血（图 6-08）：标本为大脑与脑桥的剖面。大脑出血的部位是内囊
（➡），出血处组织被破坏。

Hypertensive cerebral hemorrhage（Fig. 6-08）：The specimens are the brain and the pons. The part of the cerebral hemorrhage is the internal capsule（➡）, and the tissue at the hemorrhage is destroyed.

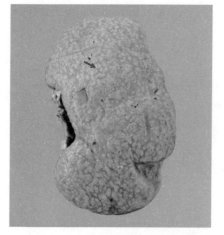

图 6-07　高血压肾病

Fig. 6-07　Hypertensive kidney

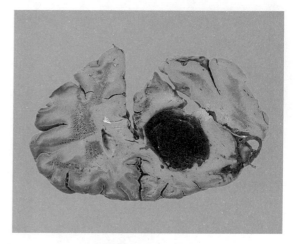

图 6-08　高血压脑出血

Fig. 6-08　Hypertensive cerebral hemorrhage

（四）风湿病及慢性心瓣膜病 Rheumatism and chronic valvular disease

（1）二尖瓣狭窄（图6-09）：二尖瓣增厚、粘连，瓣膜口狭窄如铅笔芯样（➡），左心房扩大（部分已被剪去）。右心扩大，三尖瓣无明显器质性病变，但瓣膜口相对关闭不全（★）。

思考题：此例标本左心房为何会扩大？左心室为何会缩小？

Mitral stenosis（Fig. 6-09）：The leaflet of the mitral valves thickened, hardened, and shortened, and fibrosis across the valve create "pencil lead" stenosis（➡）. The left atrium is dilated, and the left ventricular shrink. There is no obvious organic lesion in tricuspid valve, but the orifice of the valve is incompletely atretic (relatively)（★）.

Question：Why is the left atrium dilated? Why does the left ventricular shrink?

（2）二尖瓣狭窄伴左心房球形血栓（图6-10）：二尖瓣增厚、粘连，瓣膜口狭窄（➡），左心房扩大，局部左心房壁见直径2.5 cm的红褐色球形病变（★）；左心室缩小。

Mitral stenosis with left atrium thrombus（Fig. 6-10）：The mitral valve is thickened, hardened, and shortened（➡）. Local left atrial wall shows a reddish-brown globular lesion (2.5 cm in diameter)（★）; left ventricular contraction.

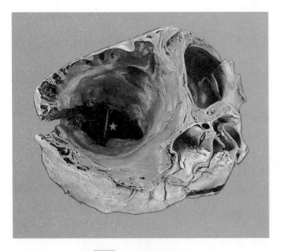 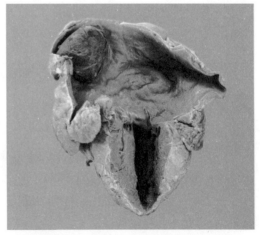

图 6-09　二尖瓣狭窄　　　　　图 6-10　二尖瓣狭窄伴左心房球形血栓
Fig. 6-09　Mitral stenosis　　　Fig. 6-10　Mitral stenosis with left atrium thrombus

（3）二尖瓣狭窄伴关闭不全（图6-11）：二尖瓣增厚、粘连，瓣膜口狭窄，呈鱼口状（➡），左心房扩大（★），左心室也明显扩大。

Mitral stenosis with mitral insufficiency（Fig. 6-11）：The mitral valve, which creates "fish mouth" stenosis（➡）, is thickened, hardened, and shortened. The left atrium is dilated（★） and the left ventricle is also significantly enlarged.

（4）二尖瓣狭窄伴三尖瓣相对关闭不全（图6-12）：二尖瓣增厚、粘连，瓣膜口狭窄，裂隙呈鱼口状（➡），左心室无明显扩大。三尖瓣正常，瓣膜口扩大，形成相对关闭不全（★），右心室扩大。

Mitral stenosis and tricuspid insufficiency（Fig. 6-12）：The mitral valve is thickened, hardened, and shortened, which creates "fish mouth" stenosis（➡）. And the left ventricular keeps normal. The tricuspid valve is regurgitation due to commissural enlarged（★）, and the right ventricular dilated.

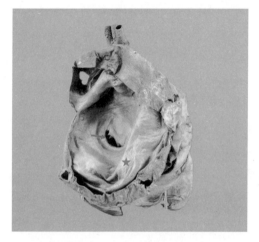 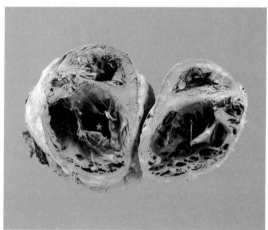

图 6-11　二尖瓣狭窄伴关闭不全　　　　　　图 6-12　二尖瓣狭窄伴三尖瓣相对关闭不全

Fig. 6-11　Mitral stenosis with mitral insufficiency　　Fig. 6-12　Mitral stenosis and tricuspid insufficiency

（四）感染性心内膜炎 Infective endocarditis

亚急性感染性心内膜炎（图 6-13）：主动脉瓣增厚，瓣膜交界处粘连，瓣膜处可见不规则、直径约 0.5 cm 的灰黄色赘生物（➡），主动脉有粥样硬化斑块。

Subacute infective endocarditis（Fig. 6-13）：The aortic valve, which is thickened and stenosis, shows an irregular, gray-yellow vegetation with a diameter of about 0.5 cm（➡）. And the valve caps are being destroyed. The surface of the aortic shows multiple yellow or grey yellow atherosclerotic plaques.

（五）心肌病 Cardiomyopathy

肥厚性心肌病（图 6-14）：以心肌肥厚为主（★），尤其是左心室室间隔明显增厚，可导致左心流出道狭窄（➡）。

Hypertrophic cardiomyopathy（Fig. 6-14）：Mainly with cardiac hypertrophy（★）, especially with obvious thickening of the left ventricular wall, which can lead to the stenosis of the left cardiac outflow tract（➡）.

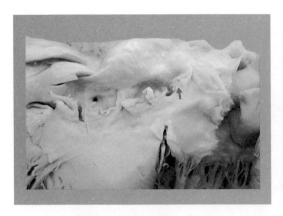

图 6-13 亚急性感染性心内膜炎
Fig. 6-13 Subacute infective endocarditis

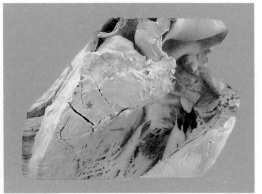

图 6-14 肥厚性心肌病
Fig. 6-14 Hypertrophic cardiomyopathy

三、组织切片观察 Observation of tissue slides

(一)动脉粥样硬化 Atherosclerosis

1. 主动脉粥样硬化 Aortic atherosclerosis (图 6-15 Fig. 6-15)

病变的内膜显著增厚、隆起,表面有纤维组织玻璃样变,为纤维帽(▲);其下方为粥样坏死灶,其中有许多呈斜方形、菱形及针形的空隙(◤)(为胆固醇结晶,在制片时被溶去后留下的空隙),有些切片可见钙化病灶;坏死灶附近尚可见许多泡沫细胞(➡),泡沫细胞体积大,呈圆形或椭圆形,胞质内含大量小空泡,细胞核位于一边或中央;中膜肌层轻度萎缩(★),外膜疏松,有少量淋巴细胞浸润。

The intima of the lesion was significantly thickened and bulge, with fibrous tissue glass-like changes on the surface, and it is a fibrous cap (▲). Beneath? the? cap, there are atheromatous foci, many of which are oblique, rhombic and needle-shaped empty? "clefts" (◤)(The space left by the dissolution of lipids in cholesterol crystals during routine production). Some sections show calcified lesions; there are still many foam cells (➡) near the necrosis, foam cells are large and round or oval shape, the cytoplasm contains a large number of small vacuoles, the nucleus is located on one side or the center; the medial muscle layer is slightly atrophic (★), the outer membrane is loose, and there is a small amount of lymphocyte infiltration.

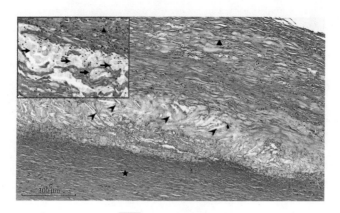

图 6-15　主动脉粥样硬化

Fig. 6-15　Aortic atherosclerosis

2. 心肌梗死 Myocardial infarction

（1）新鲜心肌梗死（图 6-16）：心外膜的冠状动脉呈偏心性狭窄（✛），内膜处可见不规则粥样硬化斑块（▲），其中有散在钙化灶（➡）；坏死的心肌细胞大部分呈凝固性坏死（◤），心肌纤维红染，细胞核消失；坏死灶周围可见充血出血炎症反应带。梗死区心内膜处可见附壁血栓（★）。

Fresh myocardial infarction（Fig. 6-16）：The epicardial coronary artery showed eccentric stenosis, and irregular atherosclerotic plaque（▲）is seen in the endocardium, in which scattered calcifications are seen（➡）. Most of the necrotic myocardial cells are coagulative necrosis（◤）, myocardial fibers are red stained, the nucleus disappear; there is congestive hemorrhagic inflammation response zone surrounding the necrosis muscle. Mural thrombus can be found in the endocardium of the infarcted area（★）.

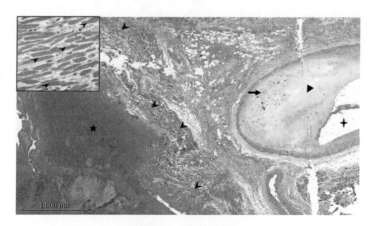

图 6-16　新鲜心肌梗死

Fig. 6-16　Fresh myocardial infarction

（2）陈旧性心肌梗死（图 6-17）：病变处仅见少量新鲜梗死灶，心肌纤维红染，横纹模糊不清,细胞核消失(➡);大多数梗死灶已被机化,在正常心肌中可见散在的纤维结缔组织(◤);梗死区心内膜可见附壁血栓(★)形成。

思考:陈旧性心肌梗死时,为什么在心肌中出现大量纤维结缔组织?

Old myocardial infarction (Fig. 6-17)：The necrotic muscles fibers are swollen, hyalinized, and lacking their striations and nuclei (➡). There is a zone of red cells surrounding pale area of necrosis muscle. Well-healed myocardial infarct with replacement of the necrotic fibers by dense collagenous scar(◤) can be found. The thrombus can be found on endocardium(★).

Question：In the case of old myocardial infarction, why is there a large amount of fibrous connective tissue in the myocardium?

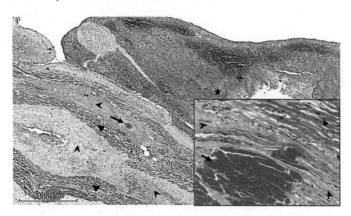

图 6-17　陈旧性心肌梗死
Fig. 6-17　Old myocardial infarction

(二) 高血压病 Hypertension

原发性细动脉硬化性固缩肾(原发性颗粒性固缩肾)(图 6-18);部分肾小球入球动脉呈均质红染的玻璃样变性,管壁增厚,管腔狭窄、闭塞(➡);小叶间动脉纤维增多,壁厚腔窄;部分肾小球纤维化,玻璃样变性(▲),相应肾小管萎缩(◤)甚至消失,间质纤维组织增生伴淋巴细胞浸润;部分肾小球代偿性肥大(★),肾小管扩张,可见均质红染的蛋白管型(✚);萎缩的肾单位与代偿性肥大的肾单位形成了颗粒状外观。

Primary contracted kidney caused by arteriosclerosis (Primary granular contracted kidney) (Fig. 6-18)：Part of the glomerular artery showed homogeneous red stained hyaline degeneration, thickening of the wall, stenosis and occlusion of the lumen (➡); the intimal fibrous tissue of interlobular artery increase and the wall thickness and lumen are narrow; some glomeruli atrophied and fibrosed(▲), and the tubule atrophied also(◤). The interstitial tissue proliferated and a few lymphocytes infiltrated. Some glomeruli are hypertrophied (★), the tubules are dilated with homogeneous red stained protein casts(✚) and atrophic nephron and compensatory hypertrophic nephron form granular appearance.

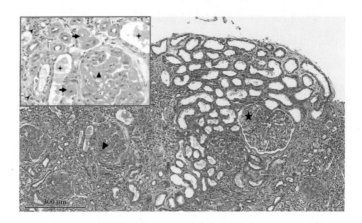

图 6-18   原发性细动脉硬化性固缩肾

Fig. 6-18   Primary contracted kidney caused by arteriosclerosis

（三）风湿病 Rheumatism

风湿性心肌炎（rheumatic myocarditis）（图 6-19）：低倍镜下，心肌（↗）间质血管（➡）附近可见呈圆形或卵圆形结节状的风湿 Aschoff 小体（★）；高倍镜下，Aschoff 小体中心尚可见红染的纤维素样坏死组织，周围为较多的风湿细胞（Aschoff 细胞）伴少量淋巴细胞、单核细胞浸润；Aschoff 细胞（▲）体积大，圆形或多边形，胞浆丰富，嗜碱性，核呈圆形或卵圆形，位于中央，单核或双核，核膜清楚，染色质集中在核中央，横切面核呈枭眼状，纵切面呈毛虫状。

Rheumatic myocarditis（Fig. 6-19）：Low power view, Aschoff bodies（★）are located interstitially in the myocardium（↗）. The Aschoff body is oval or elongated nodule, often adjacent to a small blood vessel（➡）. High power view, in the center of Aschoff bodies, red stained cellulosic necrotic tissue can be seen, surrounded by a large number of rheumatic cells（Aschoff cells）with a small number of lymphocytes and monocytes infiltration；Aschoff cells（▲）are large, round or polygonal in size, have？ abundant？ and basophil？ cytoplasm. The nucleus is round-to-ovoid in the center, monocyte or binuclear, with clear nuclear membrane with chromatin concentrated in the center of the nucleus and the nucleus are owl eyes in transverse section and caterpillars in longitudinal section.

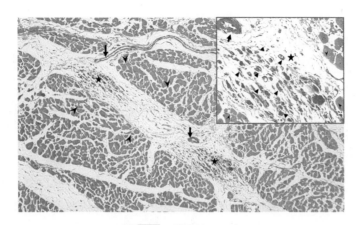

图 6-19 风湿性心肌炎

Fig. 6-19 Rheumatic myocarditis

四、 病例讨论 Case discussion

患者,女性,45 岁,因"拔牙后突发高热、呼吸困难、咳嗽、咳粉红色痰"而入院。一天前,患者因牙痛实施拔牙术,术后突发高热。入院前两个月患者曾有夜间惊醒、呼吸困难、难以平卧等症状。曾有过一次意识不清。患者 12 岁时曾患有风湿热。

体检:体温 39.5℃,心率 138 次/分,血压 90/130 mmHg。二尖瓣区可闻及收缩期吹风样杂音和舒张早期隆隆样杂音。心超检查显示二尖瓣狭窄。X 线检查显示左心房扩大、肺水肿。

思考题:结合患者的病史及临床症状、体征,你考虑该患者所患何病? 诊断依据有哪些? 患者此次与她 12 岁时所患的风湿热有关吗?

Patient, female, 45 years old. On admission to the hospital, she had high spiking fevers after undergoing a dental extraction, and she was very short of breath and had coughed up some pink frothy sputum. In one day before to her going to hospital, she went to a dentist because of tooth pain, but she had high spiking fevers after undergoing a dental extraction. In two months before hospital admission for this and related symptoms, she had awakened at night feeling short of breath. She had one fainting spell. She had history of rheumatic fever at 12-year-old.

Physical examination and laboratory tests: T 39.5℃, HR 138 times per minute, BP 90/130 mmHg. Physical examination showed turbulence produces a murmur during diastole, and producing a typical pansystolic murmur on mitral valve. Cardiac ultrasound showed narrowing of the mitral valve orifice. X-ray of her chest showed an enlarged left atrium and pulmonary edema.

Questions: What's your diagnosis? What are the diagnostic bases? Does this diagnosis have relationship with rheumatic fever at 12-year-old?

五、 思考题 Questions

（1）风湿病的基本病变是什么？

What are the basic pathological changes of rheumatic disease?

（2）各种慢性风湿性心瓣膜病有何血流动力改变及临床表现？

What are blood flow and the clinical significance of chronic rheumatic valvular heart disease?

（3）亚急性细菌性心内膜炎与风湿性心内膜炎在形态上的区别及相互关系怎样？

What are the differences and relationship between the subacute infective endocarditis and rheumatic endocarditis？

（4）冠状动脉粥样硬化的病变特点是什么？它可引起哪些严重后果？

What are pathological changes of the coronary atherosclerosis? What are complication of the coronary atherosclerosis?

（5）在高血压病晚期，心、脑、肾的病变特点及由这些病变引起的相应临床表现是什么？

What are the pathological changes and the clinical significance of heart，brain and kidney during advanced hypertension?

编写 Written by：谢芳 Xie Fang

中文审校 Chinese proofreader：邓敏 Deng Min

英文审校 English proofreader：刘瑶 Liu Yao

第七章 呼吸系统疾病

Chapter 7　Diseases of the Respiratory System

一、　教学目的 Teaching objectives

（1）熟悉慢性支气管炎及其常见并发症慢性阻塞性肺气肿和肺源性心脏病的形态学特点。

Be familiar with the morphological features of chronic bronchitis and its common complications, including chronic obstructive emphysema and chronic cor pulmonale.

（2）掌握大叶性肺炎和小叶性肺炎形态学上的基本区别。

Master the basic differences between lobar pneumonia and lobular pneumonia.

（3）熟悉支气管扩张症的形态特点。

Be familiar with the morphological features of bronchiectasis.

（4）掌握硅肺的发病机制及其主要并发症。

Master the pathogenesis of silicosis and its major complications.

（5）掌握肺癌的病理类型。

Master the pathological type of lung cancer.

二、　大体标本观察 Observation of gross specimens

（一）呼吸道和肺的炎症性疾病 Inflammatory diseases of the respiratory tract and lungs

（1）大叶性肺炎（实变期）（图7-01）：肺切面上病变肺叶呈灰白色（★）或灰黄色，结构致密；肺泡失去含气状态而为粗糙的颗粒状物质充填，实变如肝；胸膜局部有灰白色纤维素性渗出物覆盖。

Lobar pneumonia (consolidated period) (Fig. 7-01): On the cut surface of the lung, the lesion is gray (★) or yellow-gray, with dense structure. Alveoli is filling into a coarse granular material due to loss of air; the lung is consolidated, looking like liver. The pleura is covered with grayish white fibrinous exudate.

（2）大叶性肺炎伴机化（肺肉质变）（图 7-02）：肺切面上病变肺叶上半部分被致密的灰白色结缔组织所代替（★）而丧失其正常结构及功能；肺底部分肺泡内渗出物被吸收，已恢复原来的正常海绵状结构。

Organization of the lobar pneumonia（pulmonary carnification）（Fig. 7-02）：On the cut surface of the lung, the upper part of the diseased lung lobe was replaced by dense gray-white connective tissue（★）and lost its normal structure and function. The alveolar exudate in the bottom part of the lung was absorbed and restored to its original normal spongy structure.

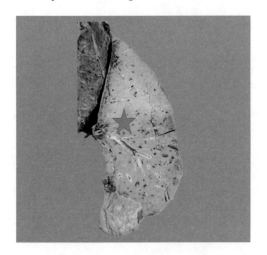

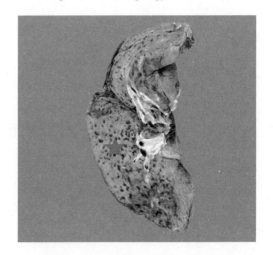

图 7-01　大叶性肺炎（实变期）

Fig. 7-01　Lobar pneumonia（consolidated period）

图 7-02　大叶性肺炎伴机化（肺肉质变）

Fig. 7-02　Lobar pneumonia with organization（pulmonary carnification）

（3）小叶性肺炎（图 7-03）：它又被称为支气管肺炎。肺切面显示典型的支气管肺炎的改变，可见沿支气管分布，呈斑片状，直径 0.3～0.5 cm 的灰黄或灰白色病灶，中央见支气管腔（➡）。

Lobular pneumonia（Fig. 7-03）：It is also known as bronchopneumonia. The cut surface of this lung demonstrates the typical appearance of bronchopneumonia. A variety of grayish or yellowish white lesions ranging in diameter of 0.3 – 0.5 cm, distributed along the bronchus, and the bronchial lumen is seen in the center（➡）.

（4）融合性小叶性肺炎（图 7-04）：儿童肺切面上显示典型的支气管肺炎，可见散在黄褐色或灰白色病变。下叶肺组织病灶已融合，形成大片突变区（★），称为融合性小叶性肺炎。

Confluent lobular pneumonia（Fig. 7-04）：The cut surface of a kid's lung demonstrates the typical appearance of a bronchopneumonia with areas of tan-yellow or gray-white lesion. These areas merged in the lower lobe, forming a consolidation（★）, called confluent lobular pneumonia.

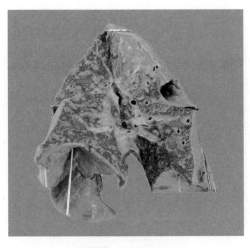

图 7-03　小叶性肺炎
Fig. 7-03　Lobular pneumonia

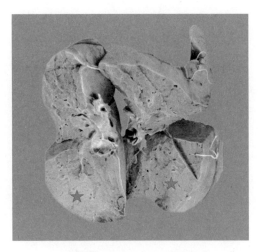

图 7-04　融合性小叶性肺炎
Fig. 7-04　Confluent lobular pneumonia

（二）慢性阻塞性肺疾病 Chronic obstructive pulmonary disease

（1）慢性支气管炎（图 7-05）：肺切面上可见到支气管纵、横断面，支气管管壁明显增厚（➡），管腔变窄，黏膜皱襞粗糙（★），少量管腔内可见淡黄色黏液脓性分泌物积聚（➡），部分肺组织呈肺气肿样改变（▲）。

Chronic bronchitis（Fig. 7-05）：The bronchial longitudinal and transverse sections are seen on the lung cut surface, and the bronchial wall is obviously thickened （➡）. The bronchial lumen is narrowed with rough mucosal folds（★）, and a few lumen is filled with pale yellow mucus purulent secretion （➡）. Some lung tissues showed emphysema （▲）.

（2）慢性支气管炎伴阻塞性肺气肿（图 7-06）：整个肺组织疏松，肺泡弥漫性膨胀，部分肺泡隔断裂，相邻肺泡腔融合成蜂窝状（➡）。标本上还可以看见慢性支气管炎表现，如支气管内黏液栓子（➡）及细支气管周围炎（▲）。

Chronic bronchitis with obstructive emphysema（Fig. 7-06）：The entire lung tissue is loose, and the alveolar diffusely expands. Part of the alveolar septum breaks , and the adjacent alveolar cavity fuses into a honeycomb （➡）, and chronic bronchitis manifestations can also be seen on the specimen, including intramucosal mucus emboli （➡） and peribronchitis （▲）.

思考题：肺气肿时，肺含气量增多，为什么患者却往往表现为缺氧？

Question：Why the patients with emphysema often have hypoxia even though there are more air in their lungs？

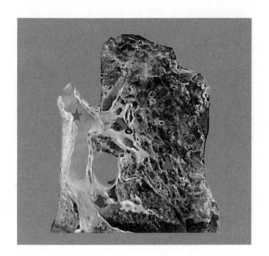 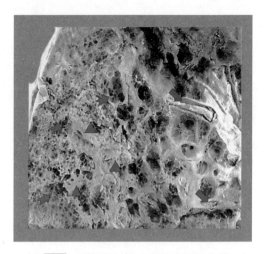

图 7-05　慢性支气管炎　　　　　　　　　图 7-06　慢性支气管炎伴阻塞性肺气肿

Fig. 7-05　Chronic bronchitis　　　　　Fig. 7-06　Chronic bronchitis with obstructive emphysema

（3）支气管扩张症（图 7-07）：肺切面上可见扩张支气管的纵、横切面或呈圆柱状，或呈囊状（➡），管壁增厚，黏膜粗糙，周围肺组织呈炎症改变。

Bronchiectasis（Fig. 7-07）: The longitudinal and transverse sections of the dilated bronchus can be seen on the lung cut surface. It can be cylindrical or saclike（➡）. The wall of the bronchus is thickened, the mucosa is rough, and the surrounding lung tissue has an inflammatory change.

（三）肺尘埃沉着症 Pneumoconiosis

（1）硅肺（图 7-08）：肺组织切面上可见肺的中下部（➡）及肺门淋巴结内（➡）较多散在的针尖大、灰白色、略具光泽的小点（硅结节）。上述变化在黑色（炭末沉着）背景处更明显。有些病灶已融合，形成大片灰白色致密区（★）；胸膜纤维性增厚（✚），叶间隔分界不清；上叶肺组织疏松，呈代偿性肺气肿改变（▲）。

Silicosis（Fig. 7-08）: On the cut surface of the lung tissue, it can be seen that there are many small tip-size spots（silicon nodules）scattered on the middle lower part of the lung（➡）and the hilar lymph node（➡）. The above changes are more obvious in the background of black（carbon deposition）. Some lesions have been fused, forming a large gray-white dense area（★）. The pleura is fibrously thickened（✚）. The division of the lobes is unclear. The upper lobe lung tissue is loose, showing compensatory emphysema（▲）.

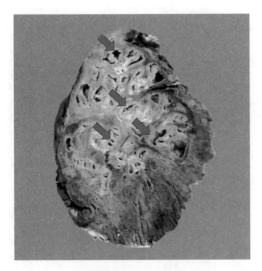

图 7-07　支气管扩张症

Fig. 7-07　Bronchiectasis

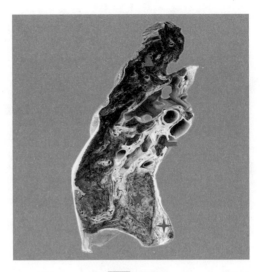

图 7-08　硅肺

Fig. 7-08　Silicosis

（2）硅肺结核（图 7-09）：硅肺病变典型，可见灰白色小结节（➡）。除此以外，尚可见大小不等的灰黄色干酪样坏死灶（结核病变）（➡），并可见大小不等的结核性空洞形成（★）。

Silicosis with tuberculosis（Fig. 7-09）：Siliceous lung lesions are typical, with grayish white nodules（➡）. In addition to the above-mentioned silicosis, there are also a number of gray-yellow caseous necrosis（tuberculosis lesions）of varying sizes（➡）, and different sizes of tuberculous cavity formation（★）.

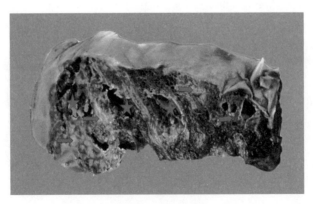

图 7-09　硅肺结核

Fig. 7-09　Silicosis with tuberculosis

思考题：硅肺最常见的并发症为结核病，为什么？

Question：Why is tuberculosis the most common complication of silicosis?

（四）慢性肺源性心脏病 Chronic cor pulmonale

慢性肺源性心脏病的心脏改变（图7-10）：在心脏横断面上，切面的空腔为右心室，小的空腔为左心室，右心室显著扩张（★），室壁亦较正常增厚（正常右心室壁厚0.3～0.4 cm）。

Heart changes in chronic cor pulmonale（Fig. 7-10）：On the cross section of the heart, the cavity of the cut surface is the right ventricle, the small cavity is the left ventricle, the right ventricle is significantly expanded（★）, and the wall is thicker than normal（normal right ventricular wall thickness is 0.3 – 0.4 cm）.

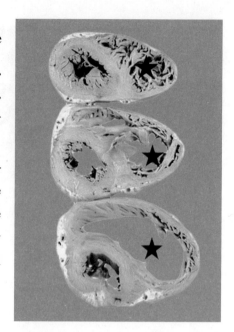

图 7-10　慢性肺源性心脏病的心脏改变
Fig. 7-10　Heart changes in chronic cor pulmonale

（五）呼吸系统肿瘤 Tumor of the respiratory system

（1）肺癌（中央型）（图7-11）：癌肿位于全肺或肺叶标本肺门处较大的支气管，并向周围肺组织浸润，形成较大的灰白色结节肿块（★）。

Carcinoma of the lung（central type）（Fig. 7-11）：The cancer is located in the larger bronchi of the hilar in the whole lung or lung lobe specimens, and infiltrated into the surrounding lung tissue, forming a large gray-white nodular mass（★）.

（2）肺癌（周围型）（图7-12）：肺周边部近胸膜处可见灰白色结节（★），结节与周围肺组织分界不清。

Carcinoma of the lung（periphery type）（Fig. 7-12）：Gray-white nodule（★）is seen near the pleura at the periphery of the lung, and the boundary between the nodules and the surrounding lung tissue was not clear.

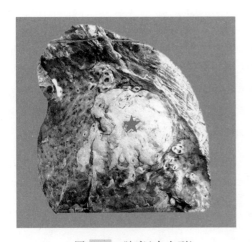

图 7-11 肺癌(中央型)

Fig. 7-11 Carcinoma of the lung (central type)

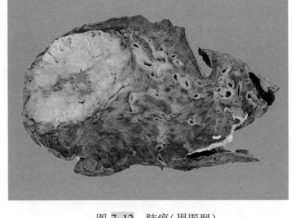

图 7-12 肺癌(周围型)

Fig. 7-12 Carcinoma of the lung (periphery type)

(3)肺癌(弥漫型)(图 7-13):癌组织呈广泛弥漫性分布。上部有较多的粟粒大、绿豆大灰白色结节(➡),中部或中下部主要为大片灰白色病变(★),与肺炎相似,临床上及病理上均须注意与肺炎区别。肺门淋巴结可见癌转移(➡)。

Carcinoma of the lung (diffuse type) (Fig. 7-13): The cancer has a wide diffuse distribution. There are more military and mung bean shaped gray nodules (➡) in the upper part. The middle or lower part is mainly a large grayish white lesion (★), which is similar to pneumonia. It needs to be

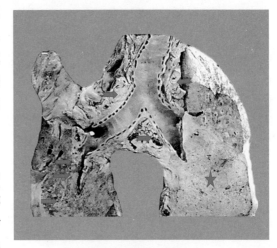

图 7-13 肺癌(弥漫型)

Fig. 7-13 Carcinoma of the lung (diffuse type)

distinguished from pneumonia both clinically and pathologically. The hilar lymph nodes showed metastasis (➡).

三、组织切片观察 Observation of tissue slides

(一)呼吸道和肺的炎症性疾病 Inflammatory diseases of the respiratory tract and lungs

(1)大叶性肺炎(图 7-14):肺泡腔充满各种渗出物,渗出物在各期有所不同,基本成分是大量纤维素(▲),此外可见大量红细胞(★)(红色肝变期)或大量中性粒细胞(◄)

（灰色肝变期）。肺泡壁毛细血管扩张充血（➡），在灰色肝变期肺泡壁毛细血管受压呈贫血状；肺泡壁结构（✚）一般未被破坏。

Lobar pneumonia（Fig. 7-14）：Most of the alveolar spaces are filled with various exudates, which are idential at different stages. Basically, the exudates are mainly cellulose（▲）, and a large number of red blood cells（★）（in the phase of red hepatization）, or a large number of neutrophils（◥）（in the phase of grey hepatization）. The capillaries of the alveolar spaces are obviously dilated and congested（➡）. In the phase of grey hepatization, the alveolar wall capillary is compressed, with fewer blood filling in. The alveolar walls are often complete（✚）.

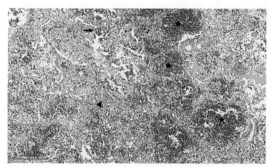 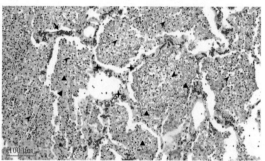

红色肝样变期 phase of red hepatization　　　灰色肝样变期 phase of gray hepatization

图 7-14　大叶性肺炎

Fig. 7-14　Lobar pneumonia

（2）小叶性肺炎（图7-15）：肺组织中可见散在病灶，病灶中央细支气管（★）管壁充血、水肿，中性粒细胞浸润，黏膜上皮（➡）坏死脱落，管腔内充满脓性渗出物（▲）；细支气管周围受累的肺泡腔内有脓性渗出物（◥）及一些红细胞、脱落的肺泡上皮细胞。严重者，病灶相互融合，呈片状分布；病灶之间的肺组织呈不同程度的代偿性肺气肿；间质血管扩张充血（✚）。

Lobular pneumonia（Fig. 7-15）：Scattered lesion can be seen in the lung tissue, with bronchioles in the central of lesions（★）, as well as congestion, edema, neutrophil infiltration, mucosal epithelial necrosis（➡）, and purulent exudates in the lumen（▲）. There are purulent exudate（◥）, some red blood cells and exfoliated alveolar epithelial cells in the alveolar space surrounding the bronchiole. In severe cases, the lesions are fused together and distributed in a sheet form. Lung tissue between the lesions show compensatory emphysema of varying degrees, and interstitial vasodilatation and hyperemia（✚）.

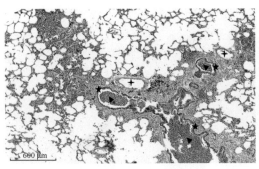 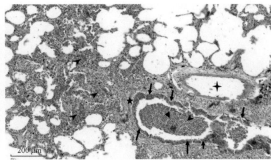

低倍镜 lower magnification　　　　　　　高倍镜 higher magnification

图 7-15　小叶性肺炎

Fig. 7-15　Lobular pneumonia

（二）慢性阻塞性肺疾病 Chronic obstructive pulmonary diseases

（1）肺气肿（图7-16）：大部分肺泡呈过度充气状态，肺泡扩大（★），肺泡间隔变窄（➡），毛细血管受压闭塞；部分肺泡间隔断裂，肺泡腔扩大形成较大囊腔（▲）；少数间质小血管壁明显增厚，管腔狭窄（◀）。

Pulmonary emphysema（Fig. 7-16）：Most of the alveoli are enlarged （★）, the alveolar space is narrowed （➡）, the capillaries are occluded, some of the alveolar septums are

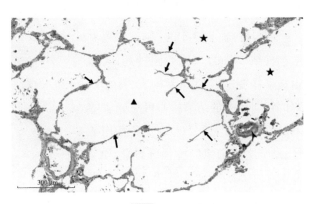

图 7-16　肺气肿

Fig. 7-16　Pulmonary emphysema

broken, and the alveolar cavity is enlarged to form a larger cyst （▲）. A small number of interstitial small vessel walls are thickened and the lumen is narrowed（◀）.

（2）支气管扩张症（图7-17）：肺内小支气管明显扩张（★），个别呈囊状，管腔内残留有黏液、炎性渗出物和红细胞（✚）；黏膜上皮增生（➡），可伴有鳞化；支气管壁平滑肌、弹力纤维、软骨遭破坏而断裂、破碎、萎缩，甚至完全消失；管壁慢性炎细胞浸润（◀）及肉芽组织形成；支气管管壁周围的肺组织萎陷、纤维化（▲）。

Bronchiectasis（Fig. 7-17）：The small bronchus in the lungs is obviously dilated （★）. Some even form cysts with mucus, inflammatory exudates and erythrocyte inside （✚）. The bronchial epithelium has mild hyperplasia（➡）（some with squamous metaplasia）. The smooth muscle, elastic fiber, and cartilage of the bronchial wall are destroyed, broken, shrunken, or even completely disappeared. Inflammatory cell infiltration （◀） and granulation are observed.

Atrophy and fibrosis of surrounding lung tissues are found around the bronchiolar walls（▲）.

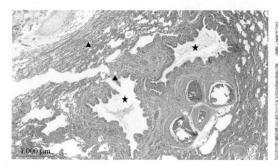
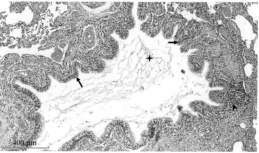

低倍镜 lower magnification　　　　　　高倍镜 higher magnification

图 7-17　支气管扩张症

Fig. 7-17　Bronchiectasis

（三）肺尘埃沉着症 Pneumoconiosis

（1）硅肺（图7-18）：肺组织可见散在硅结节（★）呈同心圆排列，大多由玻璃样变的胶原纤维构成，犹如洋葱的切面。有的结节中心可见到管壁增厚的小血管，部分硅结节已互相融合；结节之间肺组织弥漫纤维化（▲）伴少数吞噬细胞及淋巴细胞浸润（◀）；残存的肺组织呈代偿性气肿（✛）。

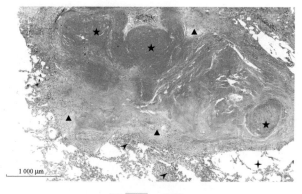

图 7-18　硅肺

Fig. 7-18　Silicosis

Silicosis（Fig. 7-18）：Most of the small nodules are visible in the section, consisting of collagen fibers arranged in concentric circles and mostly glass-like, like the cut surface of the onion, which is the silicon nodule（★）. In some centers of nodules, blood vessels with thickened walls are seen. Some of these nodules merged with others. Diffuse fibrotic focus（▲）and a few phagocgte and lymphocyte infiltrate（◀）are running in between the nodules. The remaining lung tissue has compensatory emphysema（✛）.

（四）呼吸系统肿瘤 Tumors of the respiratory system

肺鳞状细胞癌（图7-19）：癌组织（★）呈浸润性生长，破坏正常肺组织结构，与正常肺组织（▲）之间未见包膜。癌巢形态大小不一，多数癌巢的细胞排列层次与复层鳞状上皮有一定的相似之处。癌巢边缘细胞类似基底细胞，而中央细胞呈多边形，胞浆丰富，类似棘细胞。癌细胞大,异型,核分裂象多。部分癌巢中央有坏死,以致有的形成假腺样结构。本例为非角化型鳞癌。残留的肺组织有炎症反应(◀)。

Squamous cell carcinoma of the lung (Fig. 7-19): The cancer tissue (★) showed invasive growth, destroying the normal lung tissue structure, and no envelope was observed between the normal lung tissue (▲). The tumor lesions have varying sizes and

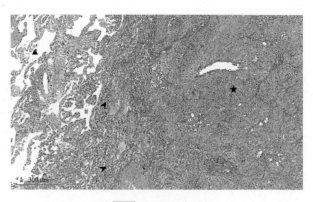

图 7-19 肺鳞状细胞癌
Fig. 7-19 Squamous cell carcinoma of the lung

shapes. The arrangement of tumor cells has some similarities with the stratified squamous epithelium. The cells in the periphery resemble basal cells, while the cells in the center are more similar to prickle cells, which are polygonal and rich in cytosol. The cancer cells are enlarged, anaplastic, and with many mitotic figures. Necrosis are present in the center of some lesions, which lead to the formation of a pseudo-adenoid structure. This case is a non-keratinized squamous cell carcinoma. The remaining lung tissue has an inflammatory response(◀).

四、病例讨论 Case discussion

男性患者,20 岁,大学生。酗酒后遭雨淋,于当天晚上突然起病,出现寒战、高热、呼吸困难、胸痛等症状,继而咳嗽,咳铁锈色痰。其家属紧急送他至当地医院就诊。

听诊:左肺下叶有大量湿性啰音;触诊:语颤增强;血常规:白细胞计数 17×10^9/L;X 线检查:左肺下叶有大片致密阴影。

入院后经抗生素治疗,患者病情好转,各种症状逐渐消失;X 线检查显示左肺下叶的大片致密阴影面积缩小 2/3,无症状后出院。冬季体检,X 线检查显示左肺下叶有约 3 cm × 2 cm 大小的不规则阴影,周围边界不清,怀疑为"支气管肺癌"。当地医院给他做左肺下叶切除术。

病理检查:肺部肿块肉眼下呈红褐色肉样,镜下显示为肉芽组织。

A 20-year old university male student was soaked through by the rain when he was drunk. That night, he suddenly had chills, high fever, difficult breathing, chest pain, and then cough with rusty phlegm. His family sent him to the local hospital for treatment.

Auscultation: A large number of moist rales was heard in the lower left lobe with increased fremitus palpation. Laboratory examination: WBC 17×10^9/L. X-ray examination: A large dense shadow was seen in the left lower lobe.

After admission to the hospital for antibiotic treatment, the condition of the patient improved, and various symptoms gradually disappeared. X-ray review showed that the dense shadow of the left lower lobe was reduced by 2/3 area. The patient was discharged for no symptoms. The student had physical examination in the coming winter. The X-ray examination showed there was an irregular shadow of about 3 cm × 2 cm in the left lower lobe, which has an unclear boundary with the surrounding tissue. According to this result, the student was suspected to have bronchial carcinoma. Left lower lobe resection is performed at the local hospital.

Pathological examination: The lesion had a reddish-brown appearance which was granulation tissue under the microscope.

分析题 Questions

（1）患者发生了什么疾病？

What is your diagnosis for this student?

（2）患者为什么会出现咳铁锈色痰？

Why did he have rusty phlegm?

（3）怀疑左肺下叶的"支气管肺癌"在手术后确诊为什么病变？是如何形成的？

What is the pathological diagnosis for the suspected lesion after surgery? What is the cause of this morphological change?

四、 思考题 Questions

（1）根据下表内容比较大叶性肺炎和小叶性肺炎的不同之处。

Please compare the differences between lobar pneumonia and lobular pneumonia according to the following table.

	大叶性肺炎 Lobar pneumonia	小叶性肺炎 Lobular pneumonia
病因 Cause		
好发年龄 Age		
病变性质 Type of pathogenesis		
病变特征 Morphology		
病程 Course of disease		
预后 Prognosis		

（2）长期慢性支气管炎可引起什么后果？

What are the consequences of chronic bronchitis?

（3）慢性支气管炎如何引起肺源性心脏病？当其患者合并新的呼吸道或肺部感染时，为何易诱发心衰？

How does chronic bronchitis cause pulmonary heart disease? Why is it easy to induce heart failure when a patient has a new respiratory or pulmonary infection?

（4）肺源性心脏病的常见原因及病理变化是什么？

What are the common causes and pathological changes of pulmonary heart disease?

（5）肺癌有哪些类型？其扩散情况如何？

What are the types of lung cancer and how do they metastasize?

编写 Written by：万珊 Wan Shan

中文审核 Chinese Proofreader：邓敏 Den Min

英文审核 English Proofreader：刘瑶 Liu Yao

8

第八章　消化系统疾病

Chapter 8　Diseases of the Digestive System

一、　教学目的 Teaching objectives

（1）掌握消化性溃疡的病理变化及其主要并发症。

Master the pathological changes and complications of peptic ulcer.

（2）掌握病毒性肝炎的基本病理变化及各型临床病理特点。

Master the basic pathological changes and the clinicopathological features of each subtype in viral hepatitis.

（3）掌握各型肝硬化的病变特点及其主要后果。

Master the pathological changes and clinical outcomes of cirrhosis.

（4）掌握食管癌、胃癌、结肠癌的肉眼形态及临床表现特点。

Master the gross features and clinical presentations of esophageal, gastric and colonic carcinoma.

（5）熟悉肝癌的病变特点。

Be familiar with morphological features of the hepatic carcinoma.

二、　大体标本观察 Observation of gross specimens

（一）消化管炎症 Inflammation of the digestive tract

（1）慢性萎缩性胃炎（图8-01）：胃黏膜壁明显变薄，皱襞变窄或消失（★）。

Chronic atrophic gastritis(Fig. 8-01)：The mucosa of stomach wall is thin and the rugal folds are narrow or disappeared(★).

（2）慢性肥厚性胃炎（图8-02）：胃黏膜肥厚，皱襞宽，如脑回状（★）。

Chronic hypertrophic gastritis（Fig. 8-02）：The mucosa of stomach wall is thick and the rugal folds are wide, similar to cerebral gyri（★）.

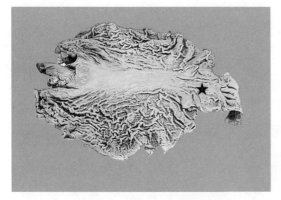

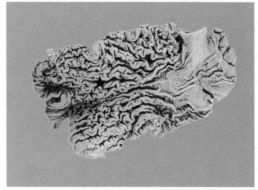

图 8-01　慢性萎缩性胃炎
Fig. 8-01　Chronic atrophic gastritis

图 8-02　慢性肥厚性胃炎
Fig. 8-02　Chronic hypertrophic gastritis

（二）慢性消化性溃疡 Chronic peptic ulcer

（1）慢性胃溃疡（图8-03）：胃小弯近幽门部有一个椭圆形的溃疡（★），溃疡直径在 2 cm 以内，边缘整齐，底部光滑。溃疡可以是单个或多发。

Chronic gastric ulcer（Fig. 8-03）：There is an oval ulcer （★）in the lesser curvature of the stomach near the pylorus. The diameter of the ulcer is within 2 cm, the edge is neat, and the bottom is smooth. The ulcer could be unifocal or multifocal.

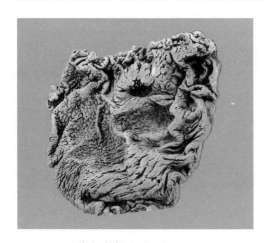

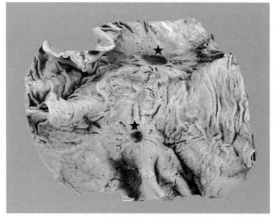

单发溃疡 single ulcer

多发溃疡 multiple ulcers

图 8-03　慢性胃溃疡
Fig. 8-03　Chronic gastric ulcer

（2）慢性十二指肠溃疡（图 8-04）：十二指肠球部黏膜面有一浅表溃疡（★），溃疡较小，直径在 1 cm 以内。

Chronic duodenal ulcer(Fig. 8-04)：There is a superficial ulcer(★) in the mucosa of the duodenal bulb，which is smaller and less than 1 cm in diameter.

（3）慢性胃溃疡伴出血（图 8-05）：溃疡底部有针孔大的血管破裂口，周围有出血，呈黑色（★）。

Chronic gastric ulcer with hemorrhage(Fig. 8-05)：At the bottom of the ulcer, there is a pinhole-sized blood vessel ruptured, and there is bleeding around it, which is black(★).

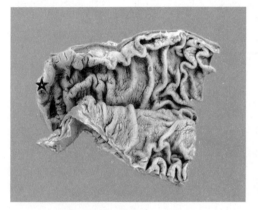 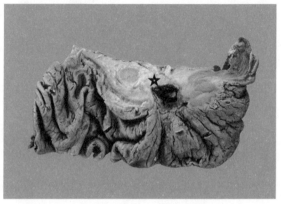

图 8-04　慢性十二指肠溃疡　　　　　　　　图 8-05　慢性胃溃疡伴出血
Fig. 8-04　Chronic duodenal ulcer　　　　Fig. 8-05　Chronic gastric ulcer with bleeding

（4）慢性胃溃疡伴慢性穿孔（图 8-06）：胃角处溃疡慢性穿孔，溃疡与胰腺粘连（★），局部胰腺组织成为溃疡底部。

Chronic gastric ulcer with chronic perforation(Fig. 8-06)：The ulcer at the angle of the stomach is chronically perforated, and it adheres to the pancreas(★). The focal pancreatic tissue becomes the base of the ulcer.

（5）慢性胃溃疡伴急性穿孔（图 8-07）：胃角处溃疡直径约 1 cm，并可见直径约 0.5 cm 的穿孔（★）。

Chronic gastric ulcer with acute perforation(Fig. 8-07)：At the angle of the stomach, there is a ulcer, 1 cm in diameter, with a perforation(★) about 0.5 cm in diameter.

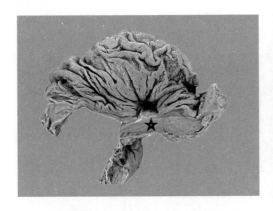

图 8-06 慢性胃溃疡伴慢性穿孔

Fig. 8-06 Chronic gastric ulcer with chronic perforation

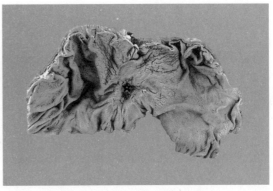

图 8-07 慢性胃溃疡伴急性穿孔

Fig. 8-07 Chronic gastric ulcer with acute perforation

（6）慢性十二指肠溃疡伴急性穿孔（图8-08）：十二指肠球部可见直径约 1 cm 的穿孔（★）。

Chronic duodenal ulcer with acute perforation（Fig. 8-08）：A perforation（★）of about 1 cm in diameter is seen in the duodenal bulb.

思考题：上消化道穿孔病人可能出现哪些临床症状或体征？如何进一步确诊？

Question：What are the clinical signs or symptoms of patients with upper gastrointestinal perforation？How to confirm the diagnosis？

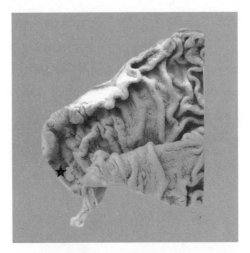

图 8-08 慢性十二指肠溃疡伴急性穿孔

Fig. 8-08 Chronic duodenal ulcer with acute perforation

（三）病毒性肝炎 Viral hepatitis

（1）急性重型病毒性肝炎（图 8-09）：成人肝脏极度缩小，包膜皱缩（图 8-09 左图 ★），边缘锐利（图 8-09 右图 ★），呈灰黄色或灰红褐色，并杂以褐色出血坏死区及暗绿色的胆汁淤结区。

Acute sever viral hepatitis（Fig. 8-09）：The size of this adult's liver is extremely reduced, with shrinking capsule, sharp edges, and grayish yellow or grayish reddish brown color. It is mixed with brown hemorrhagic necrotic area and dark green cholestasis area.

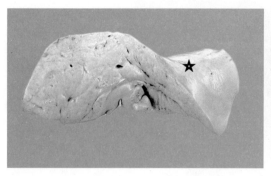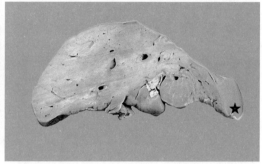

图 8-09　急性重型病毒性肝炎

Fig. 8-09　Acute severe viral hepatitis

（2）亚急性重型病毒性肝炎（图 8-10）：成人肝脏，体积明显缩小，包膜皱缩，边缘锐利，呈灰褐色，表面及切面可见散在分布的不规则的细小结节（➡），结节间为灰黄色的坏死肝组织（★）。

Subacute severe viral hepatitis（Fig. 8-10）：The volume of the adult's liver is significantly reduced, with shrinking capsule, sharp edges, and gray-brown color. Its surface and the cut surface are scattered with irregular small nodules（➡）, as well as grayish yellow necrotic liver tissue（★）.

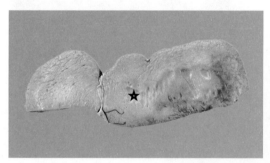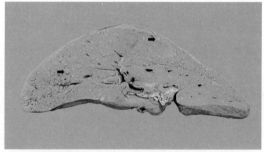

图 8-10　亚急性重型病毒性肝炎

Fig. 8-10　Subacute severe viral hepatitis

（四）肝硬化 Cirrhosis

（1）小结节性肝硬化（图 8-11）：成人肝脏，体积缩小，表面及切面有分布不均匀、大小相似的细结节（直径 0.2～1 cm，但多数较小），结节间被较窄的结缔组织所分隔。

Micronodular cirrhosis（Fig. 8-11）：The adult's liver, with a reduced volume, sees finely distributed, similarly sized nodules（0.2－1 cm in diameter, but most of them are small）. The nodules are seperated by narrow connective tissues.

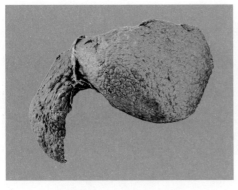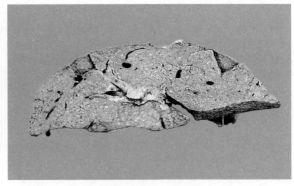

肝表面 the liver surface　　　　　　　　　　肝切面 the cut surface

图 8-11　小结节性肝硬化

Fig. 8-11　Micronodular cirrhosis

（2）大结节性肝硬化（图8-12）：成人肝脏体积缩小。肝表面及切面有分布不均匀、大小相差悬殊的粗大结节（直径0.2～2 cm，但多数较大），其间为宽窄不等的结缔组织所分隔包绕。

Macronodular cirrhosis（Fig. 8-12）：The volume of this adult's liver is reduced. Its surface and the cut surface are unevenly distributed with the large and small nodules（0.2 – 2 cm in diameter，but most of them are large），which are separated by unevenly wide and narrow connective tissues.

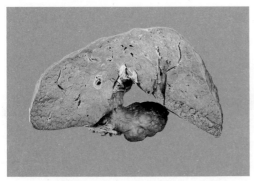

结节大小不一 nodules vary in size　　　　　　　结节粗大 larger nodules

图 8-12　大结节性肝硬化

Fig. 8-12　Macronodular cirrhosis

（3）胆汁性肝硬化（图8-13）：肝脏体积略缩小，表面呈黄绿色，可见不规则分布的细颗粒，但不如上述两型肝硬化明显。有的标本结节可见到扩张的细胆管呈网状分布，切面也呈黄绿色，汇管区结缔组织增生。

Biliary cirrhosis（Fig. 8-13）：The liver is slightly smaller in size，the surface is yellow-green，and irregularly distributed fine particles are visible，but not as obvious as the above two types of cirrhosis. Some specimen nodules can be seen that the expanded thin bile duct is distributed in a network, the cut surface is also yellow-green, and the connective tissue is proliferated in the portal area.

（4）慢性脾淤血（图 8-14）：脾脏肿大，包膜增厚，淤血（紫红色）显著，切面可见散在的芝麻大或米粒大的灰黄色结节（➡）。

Chronic splenic congestion（Fig. 8-14）：The spleen is enlarged, with thickened the capsule and remarkable congestion（purple red）. The cutting surface sees scattered seed-like or grain-like nodules（➡）.

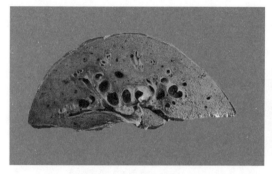 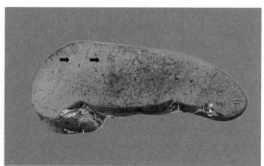

图 8-13　胆汁性肝硬化　　　　　　　　　图 8-14　慢性脾淤血

Fig. 8-13　Biliary cirrhosis　　　　　　　Fig. 8-14　Chronic spleen congestion

（5）食管黏膜下静脉曲张（图 8-15）：食管下端黏膜下静脉曲张显露（➡），局灶出血（★）。

Esophageal submucous varices（Fig. 8-15）：Submucosal varices at the lower end of the esophagus were exposed（➡），with focal bleeding（★）.

（五）消化系统肿瘤 Tumors of the digestive system

1. 食管癌 Esophageal carcinoma

（1）髓质型（图 8-16）：癌组织向食管壁浸润生长，也有向管腔内生长的趋势，故除管壁增厚外，管腔内亦可见到坡状隆起的癌组织，表面亦可形成溃疡。

Medullary type（Fig. 8-16）：The tumor infiltrates into the esophageal wall, as well as projects into the lumen. So the esophageal wall is thickened and there is a mass in the lumen, with ulceration in the surface.

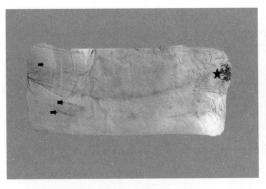

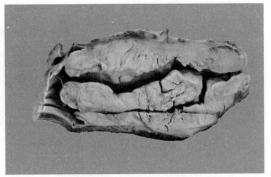

图 8-15　食管黏膜下静脉曲张

Fig. 8-15　Esophageal submucosal varices

图 8-16　食管癌(髓质型)

Fig. 8-16　Esophageal carcinoma (medullary type)

（2）蕈伞型（图 8-17）：癌组织向管腔内生长，形成蕈伞状（★），突出于管腔中。

Fungoid type（Fig. 8-17）：The tumor projects into the lumen, looking like a mushroom（★）.

（3）溃疡型（图 8-18）：癌组织向食管壁浸润生长，因癌组织的坏死脱落而形成溃疡（★），溃疡周围黏膜隆起。

Ulcerative type（Fig. 8-18）：The tumor infiltrates into the esophageal wall. Ulcer（★）is formed due to the necrosis of the fast-growing tumor and the surrounding mucosa looks like a crater.

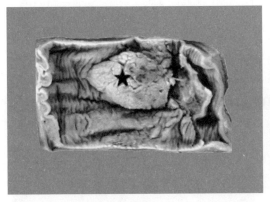

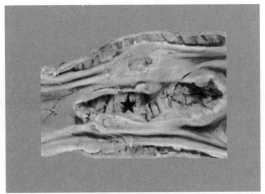

图 8-17　食管癌(蕈伞型)

Fig. 8-17　Esophageal carcinoma (fungoid type)

图 8-18　食管癌(溃疡型)

Fig. 8-18　Esophageal carcinoma (ulcerative type)

（4）缩窄型：癌组织主要浸润食管壁并环绕食管生长，使局灶食管管腔明显狭窄。

Annular type：The tumor tissue infiltrates into the wall and keeps growing surrounding the esophagus, leading the obvious narrowing of the esophageal lumen.

2. 胃癌 Gastric carcinoma

（1）息肉型（图 8-19）：肿瘤多在小弯侧，主要向胃腔内生长，形成息肉样肿块凸出于胃腔中，表面有浅表溃疡形成。

Polypoid type（Fig. 8-19）：The tumor mass often locates in the lesser curvature, projecting into the lumen, with shallow ulcer at the surface.

（2）溃疡型（图 8-20）：癌肿位于胃小弯近幽门部，呈溃疡状，直径在 2.5 cm 以上，边缘不规则，并常呈围堤状隆起。

Ulcerative type（Fig. 8-20）：The tumor locates in the lesser curvature of stomach near the pylorus. There is a ulcer in the tumor with a diameter more than 2.5 cm, raised edges, and irregular shape.

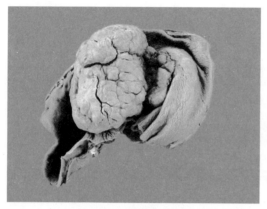

图 8-19　胃癌（息肉型）
Fig. 8-19　Gastric adenocarcinoma（polypoid type）

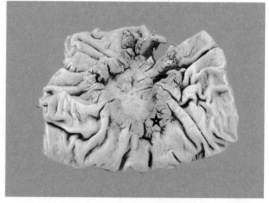

图 8-20　胃癌（溃疡型）
Fig. 8-20　Gastric adenocarcinoma（ulcerative type）

思考题：如何从肉眼上鉴别溃疡型胃癌与慢性胃溃疡病？请比较图 8-21a、b 两图，哪个是慢性胃溃疡？哪个是溃疡型胃癌？

Question：How to distinguish ulcerative gastric cancer from chronic gastric ulcer disease from the naked eye? Please compare Figure 8-21a and Figure 8-21b, which is chronic gastric ulcer? Which is ulcerative gastric cancer?

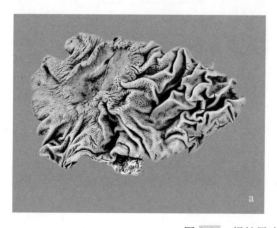
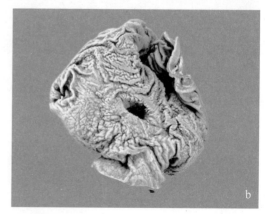

图 8-21　慢性胃溃疡与溃疡型胃癌
Fig. 8-21　Chronic gastric ulcer and ulcerative gastric cancer

（3）浸润型（图 8-22）：灰白色癌肿组织位于幽门及部分胃体部,不形成明显肿块而主要向胃壁内广泛弥漫性浸润,导致该处胃壁明显增厚。弥漫浸润时,胃壁普遍增厚、变硬,胃腔变小,形成"革囊胃"。

Infiltrative type（Fig. 8-22）: The gray-white tumor tissue locates in the pylorus and part of the gastric body, infiltrating diffusely into the stomach wall, leading to the prominent thickness of the wall. After diffuse infiltration, the stomach wall is generally thickened, hardened, and the gastric cavity becomes smaller, forming a "skin sac stomach".

（4）弥漫浸润型-胶样癌（图 8-23）：癌组织含大量黏液,呈胶冻状（★）。

Diffuse infiltrative type-colloid carcinoma（Fig. 8-23）: There are lots of mucus in the tumor, looking like jelly（★）.

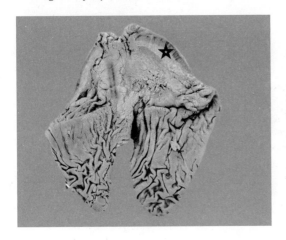 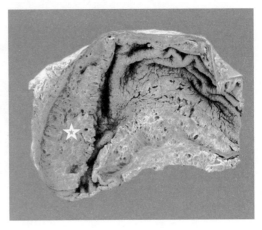

图 8-22　胃癌（浸润型）
Fig. 8-22　Gastric adenocarcinoma
（infiltrative type）

图 8-23　胃癌（弥漫浸润型-胶样癌）
Fig. 8-23　Gastric adenocarcinoma
（diffuse infiltrative type-colloid carcinoma）

3. 大肠癌 Colorectal carcinoma

请自己观察大肠癌隆起型（图 8-24）、溃疡型（图 8-25）和浸润型（图 8-26）。

Please observe the exogenous（fig. 8-24）, ulcerative（fig. 8-25）and infiltrative types（fig. 8-26）of colorectal carcinoma by yourself.

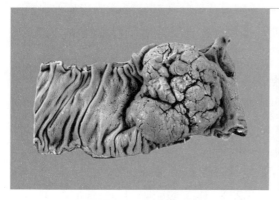

图 8-24 大肠癌（隆起型）

Fig. 8-24 Colorectal carcinoma（exogenous type）

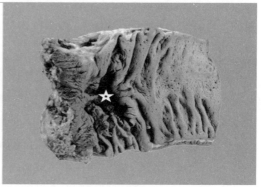

图 8-25 大肠癌（溃疡型）

Fig. 8-25 Colorectal carcinoma（ulcerative type）

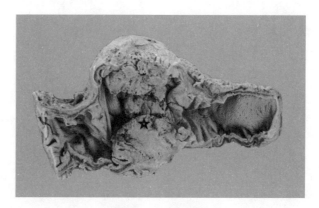

图 8-26 大肠癌（浸润型）

Fig. 8-26 Colorectal carcinoma（infiltrative type）

4. 原发性肝癌 Primary hepatic carcinoma

（1）巨块型（图 8-27）：大部分肝组织被破坏，被巨大的肿瘤结节（★）占据；各标本的肿瘤色泽不一，有的呈白色或灰红色，有的呈淡灰绿色，有的有出血、坏死或瘀胆。癌肿周围肝组织受压迫，部分标本的肝组织呈肝硬化表现。

Massive type（Fig. 8-27）：The massive nodule（★）occupies almost the entire liver. The carcinoma tissue seems gray-white, gray-red due to hemorrhagic necrosis and sometimes green due to bile retention. In addition, cirrhosis can be seen surrounding the tumor.

（2）结节型伴肝硬化（图 8-28）：有多数大小不等的灰黄色肿瘤结节（★），有的融合成较大的块状，部分标本的肝组织呈门脉性肝硬化（➡）表现。

Nodular type with cirrhosis（Fig. 8-28）：There are several tumor nodules（★）with variable size. Some nodules fused, and some area showed cirrhotic（➡）change.

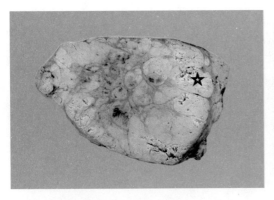

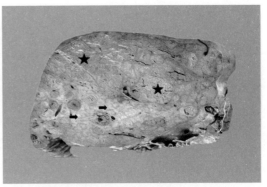

图 8-27　肝癌(巨块型)　　　　　　　　图 8-28　肝癌(结节型伴肝硬化)

Fig. 8-27　Hepatic carcinoma (massive 　　Fig. 8-28　Hepatic carcinoma (nodular

type with cirrhosis)　　　　　　　　　　　　type with cirrhosis)

思考题:肝癌的临床表现有哪些? 其肝脏往往伴有什么病变?

Question:What are the clinical presentations of liver cancer? Which diseases could often co-

exist?

三、 组织切片观察 Observation of tissue slides

(1) 慢性浅表性胃炎(图 8-29):炎症主要限于黏膜浅层,固有膜(▲)中可见淋巴细胞
和浆细胞等慢性炎细胞浸润(◀),没有固有腺体的萎缩。★示黏膜肌层。

Chronic superficial gastritis(Fig. 8-29): Inflammation is mainly limited to the superficial
mucosa. In the lamina proporia (▲), chronic inflammatory cells such as lymphocytes and
plasma cells are infiltrated (◀), and there is no atrophy of the intrinsic gland. Mucosal muscle
layer is marked by ★.

(2) 慢性萎缩性胃炎(图 8-30):胃黏膜节段性萎缩,胃小凹变浅(➡);固有膜腺体数
量减少,体积缩小(▲),并有肠上皮化生及慢性炎性细胞浸润,淋巴滤泡形成(★);固有膜
纤维组织增生。

Chronic atrophic gastritis(Fig. 8-30): The gastirc mucosa shows segmental atrophy with
shallow stomach pit (➡). The number and volume of intrinsic glands are reduced (▲), with
the presence of intestinal metaplasia. There are chronic inflammatory cells infiltration, lymphoid
follicle formation (★), and fibrous tissue hyperplasia in the lamina propria.

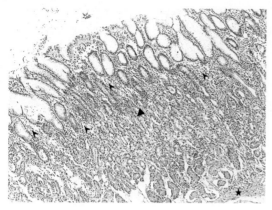

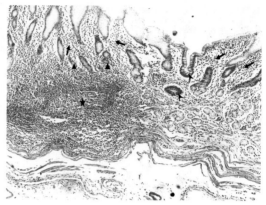

图 8-29　慢性浅表性胃炎

Fig. 8-29　Chronic superficial gastritis

图 8-30　慢性萎缩性胃炎

Fig. 8-30　Chronic atrophic gastritis

（3）慢性消化性胃溃疡（图 8-31）：胃壁局部黏膜层、黏膜下层、肌层已完全被破坏，形成溃疡。溃疡底从内到外可见四层结构，它们分别是：① 渗出层（➡）：炎性渗出物，主要为中性粒细胞及纤维素。② 坏死层（▲）：为伊红染色、结构不清的组织，混有一些破碎的细胞核。③ 肉芽组织层（◀）：为丰富的新生毛细血管、成纤维细胞，并有较多的炎症细胞浸润。④ 瘢痕层（✚）：为胶原纤维组织，血管较少。有时可见管壁增厚、管腔狭窄的厚壁血管（★）。

Chronic gastric ulcer（Fig. 8-31）：The ulcer destroyed the local mucosal layer, submucosa and muscle layer of the stomach wall. The bottom of the ulcer can be seen in four layers from the inside to the outside, which are：① Exudation layer （➡）：Inflammatory exudates, mainly neutrophils and cellulose. ② Necrotic layer （▲）：The tissue with unclear structure of eosin staining, mixed with some broken nuclei. ③ Granulation tissue layer （◀）：rich in newborn capillaries, fibroblasts, and more inflammatory cell infiltration. ④ Scar layer （✚）：It is a collagen fibrous tissue with few blood vessels. Sometimes thick blood vessels with thickened walls and narrow lumens can be seen （★）.

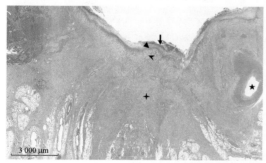

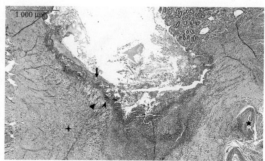

图 8-31　慢性消化性胃溃疡

Fig. 8-31　Chronic gastric ulcer

（4）病毒性肝炎（图8-32）：主要观察病毒性肝炎的基本病变。① 细胞水肿：肝细胞体积增大，部分肝细胞肿大呈球形，胞浆疏松而淡染，胞核固缩（➡）。② 嗜酸性变（◀）：肝细胞核固缩，胞浆红染。③ 脂肪变性（⇛）。④ 嗜酸性小体：无结构的、均质状的伊红色球状小体（体积相当于红细胞的 3 ~ 4 倍以上），多数已脱入肝窦内。⑤ 肝细胞点状坏死（◀◀）：坏死的肝细胞轮廓不清或消失。⑥ 肝细胞再生（★）：肝细胞体积增大，核也增大，着色深，有的有双核。⑦ 炎症细胞浸润及 Kupper 细胞增生：坏死区机会管区内有以单核细胞及淋巴细胞为主的炎症细胞浸润；窦内 Kupper 细胞数量增加。⑧ 毛玻璃样肝细胞（▲）：肝细胞胞浆内可见淡红色细颗粒状物。

Viral hepatitis（Fig. 8-32）：Mainly observe the basic pathological changes of viral hepatitis： ① Cellular edema：The volume of hepatocytes increases, and some hepatocytes become spherical with loose and empty cytoplasm and pyknotic nucleus（➡）. ② Eosinophilic change（◀）：The hepatocytic cytoplasm is red and the nucleus is pyknotic. ③ Steatosis（⇛）. ④ Eosinophilic body：Most unstructured, homogeneous eosinophilic bodies（equivalent to 3 – 4 times more than red blood cells）, fall into the liver sinus. ⑤ Hepatocyte spotted necrosis（◀◀）：The outline of necrotic hepatocytes is unclear or disappeared. ⑥ Hepatocyte regeneration（★）：The hepatocyte volume increases, the nucleus also increases, the coloration is deep, and some have a dual core. ⑦ Infiltration of inflammatory cells and proliferation of Kupper cells：Infiltration of inflammatory cells mainly composed of monocytes and lymphocytes in the necrotic area. The number of Kupper cells in the sinus increased. ⑧ Ground-glass-like hepatocytes（▲）：Light red fine particles appear in the cytoplasm of hepatocytes.

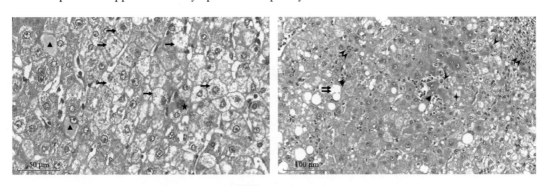

图 8-32　病毒性肝炎
Fig. 8-32　Viral hepatitis

（4）急性重型肝炎（图8-33）：大量肝细胞坏死，肝板解离，仅留细胞残影（★），肝小叶结构消失；淤胆严重，胆汁浓集成胆栓（➡），被染成金黄色的圆形团块。

Acute severe hepatitis（Fig. 8-33）：A large number of liver cells are necrotic, the liver plate dissociates, leaving only the residual image of the cells（★）, the structure of the hepatic lobule disappears. The biliary retension is severe. The bile is concentrated with the biliary plug（➡）, and it is dyed into a golden yellow round mass.

（5）亚急性重型肝炎（图8-34）：肝细胞呈亚大块坏死、消失、网状支架塌陷（★），小叶内可见少量肝细胞残留伴有多量淋巴细胞和单核细胞浸润（➡）；残存的肝细胞明显增生，增生的肝细胞常相聚成团，形成大小不等的圆形再生结节（▲），结节中的肝细胞有变性、坏死；小胆管明显增生（◀）伴扩张、淤胆。

Subacute severe hepatitis （Fig. 8-34）：Hepatocytes showed sub-macro necrosis and disappearance，and the reticular scaffold collapsed （★）. A small amount of hepatocytes remained in the lobules with a large amount of lymphocytes and mononuclear cells infiltrating （➡）. Residual hepatocytes are obviously proliferated，and proliferating hepatocytes often clustered of varying sizes. The hepatocytes in the nodules are degenerated and necrotic. The small bile ducts are obviously proliferated （◀）with dilatation and cholestatic.

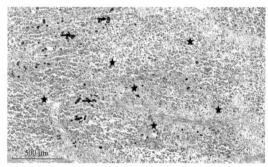
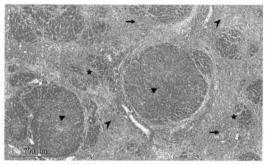

图 8-33　急性重症肝炎　　　　　　　　图 8-34　亚急性重症肝炎
Fig. 8-33　Acute severe hepatitis　　　　Fig. 8-34　Subacute severe hepatitis

（6）小结节性肝硬化（图8-35）：肝脏正常肝小叶结构被破坏并被大量假小叶（★）所取代；假小叶被肝细胞团块周围完整的、较为狭窄的纤维组织间隔（◀）围绕；其中肝细胞排列紊乱，不呈放射状，其中央静脉偏位，或有数个，或缺如；纤维组织间隔中有淋巴细胞、单核细胞浸润及小胆管增生（➡）。

Micronodular cirrhosis （Fig. 8-35）：The normal hepatic lobule structure of the liver is destroyed and replaced by a large number of pseudolobules （★）. The pseudolobules are surrounded by intact narrow fibrous tissue （◀）around the hepatocyte mass. Hepatocytes are disorderly arranged，not as radial as normal，with central venous deviation，or irregular numbers. lymphocytes and mononuclear cells infiltration，and small bile duct hyperplasia could also be seen （➡）.

（7）大结节性肝硬化（图8-36）：与小结节性肝硬化相比，假小叶大小不等（★），肝细胞变性、坏死更为明显；周围的纤维间隔宽窄不一（◀），大部分比较宽，伴有大量炎症细胞浸润和小胆管增生（➡）。

Macronodular cirrhosis（Fig. 8-36）：Compared with small nodular cirrhosis，the size of pseudolobules(★) is different, hepatocyte degeneration and necrosis are more obvious. The surrounding fiber spacing is wide and narrow (↗), and most of them are wide accompanied by a large number of inflammatory cell infiltration and small bile ducts hyperplasia (→).

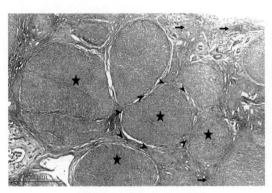

图 8-35　小结节性肝硬化
Fig. 8-35　Micronodular cirrhosis

图 8-36　大结节性肝硬化
Fig. 8-36　Macronodular cirrhosis

（7）肠腺癌及肝细胞肝癌：见第五章（肿瘤）。

Intestinal adenocarcinoma and hepatocellular carcinoma：See the description of Chapter 5 （Tumors）。

（8）请描述胃腺癌（图 8-37）组织切片的镜下表现，并根据浸润深度判断肿瘤的分期。

Please describe the section of gastric adenocarcinoma(Fig. 8-37), and determine the stage of the tumor according to the depth of infiltration.

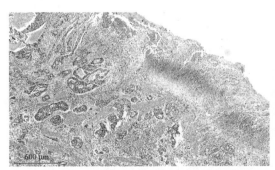
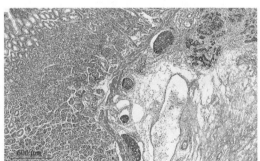

图 8-37　胃腺癌
Fig. 8-37　Gastric adenocarcinoma

思考题：消化道早期癌的判断标准是什么？

Question：How to define early gastrointestinal carcinoma？

四、 病例讨论 Case discussion

（一）病例一 Case one

患者,男,30 岁,教师。因"周期性节律性上腹部疼痛 3 年,突然剧烈疼痛伴呕吐 1 小时"入院。

患者自 3 年前开始每年天气转冷季节就发生上腹部隐痛,天气转暖后缓解,疼痛多发生在上午 11:00 左右及下午 4:00—5:00,进食后缓解,常有夜间疼痛。有时有反酸、胃烧灼感。入院当日患者中餐后突然上腹部剧烈疼痛,伴恶心、呕吐,吐出胃内容物,急诊入院。半年前曾做胃镜检查,检查结果显示十二指肠球部溃疡,溃疡灶呈椭圆形,中心覆盖白苔,周围潮红,有炎性水肿。

入院体检:体温 37.4 ℃,脉率 98 次/分,呼吸 23 次/分,血压 124/80 mmHg。急性病容,板状腹,腹部弥漫性压痛,有反跳痛。

实验室检查:白细胞计数 14.0×10^9/L,中性粒细胞 0.85;腹部 X 线透视显示膈下有游离气体。患者经外科急诊手术后治愈出院。

A 30-year-old male, who was a teacher, had periodic rhythmic upper abdominal pain for 3 years, and was admitted to hospital due to sudden severe pain with vomiting one hour ago.

The patient had the upper abdomen pain every year when the weather turned cold and lasted for three years. After the weather turned warm, the pain was relieved. The pain occurred mostly at around 11:00 am, or 4:00 − 5:00 pm, and it eased after eating. Sometimes there was acid reflux and a burning sensation in the stomach. On the day of admission, he suddenly suffered severe pain in the upper abdomen, accompanied by nausea and vomiting. He spited out stomach contents, and was admitted to the emergency room. Half a year ago, he had a gastric endoscopic examination and found a duodenal ulcer, which was oval, with white moss covered in the center, and flushing red and inflammatory edema at the periphery region.

Physical examination: Temperature 37.4 ℃, pulse rate 98 times per minute, breathing 23 times per minute, blood pressure 124/80 mmHg. The patient showed acute disease face, platy abdomen, and diffuse abdominal tenderness with rebound pain.

Laboratory examination: White blood cell count 14.0×10^9/L, neutrophils accounted 85%. Abdominal X-ray showed free gas under the diaphragm. He was cured by emergent surgery.

分析题 Questions

（1）该病人所患何病? 请说明诊断依据。

What is the disease of the patient? Please explain your diagnostic basis.

（2）请描述消化性溃疡病的病理变化、临床表现及其并发症。

Please describe the pathological changes, clinical manifestations and complications of peptic ulcer disease.

（二）病例二 Case two

患者，男，61 岁，退休工人。因"突然呕血 1 小时"入院。

患者 1 小时前进食晚餐后出现恶心，呕出鲜红色血液，量约 300 mL，无血凝块。伴头晕、心悸、口干等症状。入院后又呕鲜血约 500 mL，头昏、乏力。次晨解柏油样便 2 次，每次约 150 g。患者有乙肝病史多年，确诊"肝硬化"1 年余。

入院体检：体温 36.9 ℃，脉率 80 次/分，呼吸 22 次/分，血压 105/70 mmHg，慢性病容，颈侧见两处蜘蛛痣，巩膜无黄染，有肝掌，腹膨软，肝肋下未及，脾肋下 3 cm，腹部移动性浊音阳性。

实验室检查：总蛋白 48.1 g/L，白蛋白 27.6 g/L，球蛋白 20.5 g/L，白蛋白与球蛋白比值（A/G）为 1.3，总胆红素 27.9 μmol/L，直接胆红素 8.5 μmol/L，谷丙转氨酶 120 U/L，尿素氮 8.10 mmol/L，肌酐 120 μmol/L，葡萄糖 7.60 mmol/L。乙肝标志物测定（ELISA 法）：HBsAg 阳性、HBcAg 阳性、抗 HBc 阳性。胃镜检查显示食管中下段静脉中重度曲张。

B 超提示肝硬化、门静脉高压、脾肿大、中等量腹水。腹水常规检查显示为漏出液。腹水病理检查：未见癌细胞。患者住院后因再次大出血抢救无效而死亡。

A 61-year-old male, who was a retired worker. He was admitted to the hospital for sudden hematemesis one hour ago.

The patient developed nausea one hour after dinner, and vomited about 300 mL bright red blood without clot. He also had dizziness, palpitations, and dry mouth. After admission, he also vomited about 500 mL blood, with dizziness, and fatigue. The next morning, the patient had a total of about 150 g tarry stool. The patient had a history of hepatitis B for many years and has been diagnosed with "cirrhosis" for more than 1 year.

Physical examination: Body temperature 36.9 ℃, pulse rate 80 times per minute, breathing 22 times per minute, blood pressure 105/70 mmHg, and chronic-diseased face. The spider nevi were observed at the neck side. The patient had clear sclera, liver palms, and distended and soft abdomen. The liver could not be touched under the ribs, while the spleen was 3 cm under the ribs. Positive abdomen moving sound was also found.

Laboratory examination: Total protein 48.1 g/L, albumin 27.6 g/L, globulin 20.5 g/L, A/G ratio 1.3, total bilirubin 27.9 μmol/L, direct bilirubin 8.5 μmol/L, glutamic-pyruvic transaminase 120 U/L, urea nitrogen 8.10 mmol/L, creatinine 120 μmol/L, glucose 7.60 mmol/L. Hepatitis B serum marker assay (ELISA): HBsAg positive, HBcAg positive, anti-HBc positive. Gastroendoscope showed severe varicose veins in the middle-lower segment of the esophagus.

Ultrasound B suggesting cirrhosis, portal hypertension, splenomegaly, and moderate ascites. Ascites belongs to transudates. Ascites pathology：No cancer cells were seen. After hospitalization, he died due to repeated massive bleeding.

分析题 Questions

（1）请根据病史及检查结果做出诊断，并提供诊断依据。

Please make a diagnosis and provide a diagnosis basis based on the medical history and the results of the examination.

（2）肝硬化的病理变化是什么？请描述其临床症状与病理变化之间的联系。

What is the pathological change of cirrhosis? Please describe the correlation between clinic symptoms and pathology changes.

五、 思考题 Questions

（1）根据胃溃疡的病理形态特点，你认为溃疡不易愈合的原因是什么？它有哪些常见的并发症？

According to the pathological features of gastric ulcer, what do you think is the reason why ulcers are not easy to heal? What are the common complications?

（2）各型病毒性肝炎的病理变化有什么特点？试讨论其临床表现的病变基础。

What are the characteristics of pathological changes in various types of viral hepatitis? Try to discuss the pathological basis of clinical manifestations.

（3）试述肝炎、肝硬化和肝细胞癌之间的关系。

Describe the relationship between hepatitis, cirrhosis and hepatocellular carcinoma.

（4）根据消化道肿瘤的病理表现说明消化道肿瘤可能出现哪些临床症状。

Describe the clinical symptoms that may occur based on the pathological manifestations of digestive tract tumors.

（5）试将慢性胃溃疡与溃疡型胃癌按下表内容进行比较。

Compare chronic gastric ulcer with ulcerative gastric cancer according to the table below.

	良性溃疡（慢性消化性胃溃疡） Benign ulcer (chronic digestive gastric ulcer)	恶性溃疡（溃疡型胃癌） Malignant ulcer (ulcerative gastric cancer)
溃疡形状 Ulcer shape		
溃疡大小 Ulcer size		

续表

	良性溃疡(慢性消化性胃溃疡) Benign ulcer（chronic digestive gastric ulcer）	恶性溃疡(溃疡型胃癌) Malignant ulcer（ulcerative gastric cancer）
溃疡深度 Ulcer depth		
溃疡边缘 Ulcer edge		
溃疡底部 Ulcer base		
周围黏膜 Surrounding mucosa		

（6）请描述肝硬化病人的临床病理联系。

Please describe the correlation between clinic symptoms and pathology changes in cirrhosis.

编写 Written by：刘瑶 Liu Yao

中文审校 Chinese proofreader：邓敏 Deng Min

英文审校 English proofreader：刘瑶 Liu Yao

第九章 淋巴造血系统疾病

Chapter 9 Disorders of the Hematopoietic and Lymphoid System

一、 教学目的 Teaching objectives

（1）掌握淋巴组织肿瘤的类型及特征。

Master the types and characteristics of lymphoma.

（2）掌握霍奇金淋巴瘤与非霍奇金淋巴瘤的主要病理变化。

Master the morphologic changes of Hodgkin's and non-Hodgkin's lymphoma.

（3）熟悉白血病的主要病理变化。

Be familiar with morphologic changes of leukemia.

二、 大体标本观察 Observation of gross specimens

（一）恶性淋巴瘤 Malignant lymphoma

（1）小肠恶性淋巴瘤（图 9-01）：部分肠壁可见多灶、淡红色或灰白色、均质的鱼肉样肿瘤组织（➡）。

Malignant lymphoma of the small intestine（Fig. 9-01）：Some of the intestinal wall showed multi-focal reddish or grayish white, homogeneous fish-like tumor tissues（➡）.

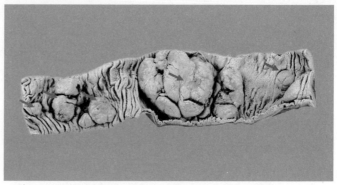

图 9-01 小肠恶性淋巴瘤

Fig. 9-01 Malignant lymphoma of the small intestine

（2）纵隔恶性淋巴瘤（图9-02）：淋巴结因肿瘤生长而增大，并互相融合成巨大肿块（➡），切面可见肿瘤呈均质、灰白色鱼肉样外观。

Malignant lymphoma of the mediastinum（Fig. 9-02）：The lymph nodes are enlarged due to tumor growth and merge into each other into a huge mass（➡）. The cut surface shows a homogeneous gray-white fish-like appearance.

（二）髓系肿瘤

慢性粒细胞性白血病的脾脏（图9-03）：脾脏高度肿大，切面呈暗红色（★），正常脾小体消失。

The spleen involved by chronic myelogenous leukemia（Fig. 9-03）：The spleen is highly enlarged, the cut surface is dark red（★）, which can't find normal structure.

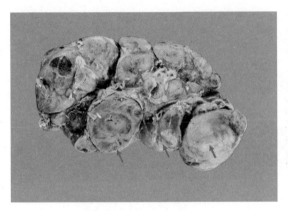

图 9-02 纵隔恶性淋巴瘤
Fig. 9-02 Malignant lymphoma of the mediastinum

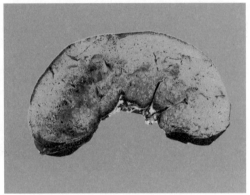

图 9-03 慢性粒细胞性白血病的脾脏
Fig. 9-03 The spleen involved by chronic myelogenous leukemia

三、 组织切片观察 Observation of tissue slides

恶性淋巴瘤 Malignant lymphoma

（1）滤泡性淋巴瘤（图9-04）：淋巴结正常结构被破坏并被肿瘤组织所替代。在弥漫分布的瘤组织中，部分区域可见瘤细胞聚集成不规则的"滤泡"样结构（◤）。瘤细胞来源于B细胞，有两种瘤细胞：①中心细胞：瘤细胞大小不等，形态不规则，核型不规则，核仁不明显；②中心母细胞：体积比较大，比正常淋巴细胞大2~3倍，核呈圆形或卵圆形，可见2~3个核仁。此外，有少量小淋巴细胞掺杂，核分裂和病理性核分裂多见。

Follicular lymphoma（Fig. 9-04）：The lymph node architecture is destroyed and replaced by tumor tissues. In diffusely distributed tumor tissue, tumor cells can be aggregated into irregular "follicle"-like structures in some areas (➹). The tumor cells resemble normal germinal center B cells. There are two manifestations of tumor cells: ① Central cells: Tumor cells vary in size, irregular shape, irregular karyotype, and nucleoli are not obvious; ② Centeroblasts: Large in size, larger than normal lymphocytes 2 – 3 times, nuclear round or oval, 2 – 3 visible nucleoli. In addition, a small number of small lymphocytes are doped, and nuclear division and pathological nuclear division are common.

（2）霍奇金淋巴瘤（混合细胞型）（图9-05）：淋巴结正常结构被破坏，瘤细胞与各种炎症细胞混合存在（炎症细胞有淋巴细胞、组织细胞、嗜酸粒细胞及浆细胞等，以小淋巴细胞为主），肿瘤以诊断性 R-S 细胞和单核型 R-S 细胞(➹)多见。R-S 细胞体积较大，胞浆丰富，核大，胞核呈圆形或卵圆形，单核或多核，核膜较厚，核仁较大，与红细胞体积相似，嗜酸性，核仁周围有空晕。双核并列似镜影，称"镜影细胞"（诊断性 R-S 细胞)(➡)。

Hodgkin's lymphoma (mixed cellularity) (Fig. 9-05): The normal structure of the lymph nodes is destroyed, and the tumor cells are mixed with various inflammatory cells (inflammatory cells include lymphocytes, histiocytes, eosinophils, and plasma cells, mainly small lymphocytes). There are many diagnostic R-S cells and mononuclear R-S cells (➹) in the tumor. R-S cells are large in volume, rich in cytoplasm, large in nucleus, round or oval in nucleus, mononuclear or multinuclear, thick nuclear membrane, large nucleoli, which is similar in volume to red blood cells, eosinophilic, and with halo around. The binuclear is like a mirror, called "mirror cells" (diagnostic R-S cells) (➡).

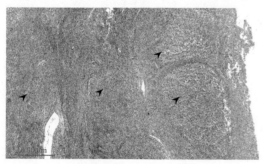

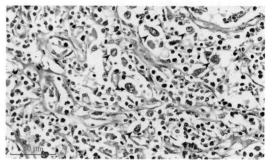

图 9-04　滤泡性淋巴瘤

Fig. 9-04　Follicular lymphoma

图 9-05　霍奇金淋巴瘤（混合细胞型）

Fig. 9-05　Hodgkin's lymphoma (mixed cellular type)

四、　病例讨论 Case discussion

患者，男，22 岁，以"发热、盗汗、体重减轻"为主诉入院。

体检：颈部淋巴结和锁骨上淋巴结肿大，淋巴结尚可活动，为无痛性。

淋巴结活检：镜下见淋巴结结构消失，细胞成分多样，有大量嗜酸粒细胞、浆细胞、组织细胞、淋巴细胞和少量中性粒细胞浸润,并有多种瘤巨细胞,体积大,呈椭圆形或不规则形;胞浆丰富,双色性或嗜酸性;核大,核内有一嗜酸性核仁,周围有一透明晕。

分析题:请对该患者做出病理诊断,并提供诊断依据。

The patient, a 22-year-old man, was admitted with fever, night sweat and weight loss.

Physical examination: Cervical lymph nodes and supraclavicular lymph nodes are swollen, movable, and painless.

Lymph node biopsy showed that the structure of lymph node disappeared, and the cell composition was diverse. There were a large number of eosinophils, plasma cells, histiocytes, lymphocytes and a small number of neutrophils infiltrated, and there were many kinds of giant tumour cells, large in size, oval or irregular. The cytoplasm was rich, bicolor eosinophilic. Large nucleus with an eosinophilic nucleolus is surrounded by a transparent halo.

Question: Please make a pathological diagnosis of the disease and provide the basis.

五、 思考题 Questions

(1)霍奇金淋巴瘤分几型? 各型病变特点及其与预后的关系如何?

How many types of Hodgkin's lymphoma? What are the characteristics of various types of lesions and their relationship with prognosis?

(2)试述弥漫性大 B 细胞淋巴瘤、滤泡性淋巴瘤的临床病理特点。

Describe the clinicopathological features of diffuse large B-cell lymphoma and follicular lymphoma.

(3)名词解释:R-S 细胞、镜影细胞、Burkitt 淋巴瘤、绿色瘤。

Definition: Reed-Sternberg cells, mirror cells, Burkitt lymphoma, chloroma.

编写 Written by:谢芳 Xie Fang
中文审校 Chinese proofreader:邓敏 Deng Min
英文审校 English proofreader:刘瑶 Liu Yao

10

第十章 泌尿系统疾病

Chapter 10　Diseases of the Urinary System

一、 教学目的 Teaching objectives

（1）掌握各型肾小球肾炎的病理特点与临床主要症状的联系。

Master the relationship between the pathological features of various types of glomerulonephritis and the main clinical symptoms.

（2）熟悉肾盂肾炎与肾小球肾炎病变的不同点。

Be familiar with the difference between pyelonephritis and glomerulonephritis lesions.

（3）了解肾癌与膀胱癌的病变特点。

Understand the pathological features of kidney cancer and bladder cancer.

二、 大体标本观察 Observation of gross specimens

（一）肾小球肾炎 Glomerulonephritis

（1）急性弥漫增生性肾小球肾炎（图 10-01）：肾体积增大。表面（图 10-01a）及切面（图 10-01b）均可见充血，呈灰红色。切面皮质增厚，髓放线肿胀、模糊不清，并可见红色小出血点，故又称"蚤咬肾"。

Acute diffuse proliferative glomerulonephritis（Fig. 10-01）：The kidney volume is increased. Its surface（Fig. 10-01a）and the cut surface（Fig. 10-01b）are both congested, with grayish red color. The cut surface cortex is thickened, and the swelling medullary line is blurred. And it can be seen that there are red small bleeding points, so the disease is also called "bite kidney".

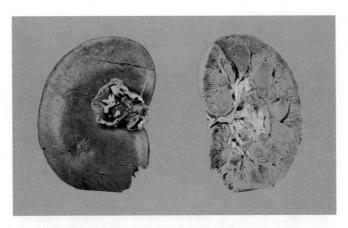

a. 表面 the surface　　　　b. 切面 the cut surface

图 10-01　急性弥漫增生性肾小球肾炎

Fig. 10-01　Acute diffuse proliferative glomerulonephritis

（2）膜性肾病（图 10-02）：肾体积增大，表面光滑呈淡黄白色，切面皮质增厚，髓放线模糊不清，又称"大白肾"。

Membranous nephropathy（Fig. 10-02）：The kidney volume is increased，the surface is smooth yellowish white，the cut surface cortex is thickened，and the medullary line is blurred. It is also known as "big white kidney".

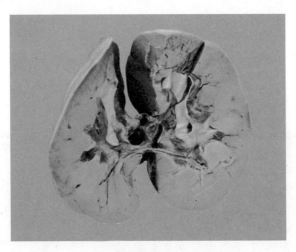

图 10-02　膜性肾病

Fig. 10-02　Membranous nephropathy

（3）慢性肾小球肾炎（图 10-03）：成人肾脏体积明显缩小，表面呈颗粒状（➡）。切面皮质变薄，皮质与髓质分界不清（✚），肾窦扩大，脂肪组织增多（➡），又称"继发性固缩肾"。

Chronic glomerulonephritis（Fig. 10-03）：The volume of adult's kidneys is significantly reduced with granular surface（➡）. In the cut surface，the cortex is thin and the demarcation between cortex and medulla is not clear （✚）. The renal sinus is enlarged and the adipose tissue is increased （➡）, It is also known as "secondary pyknosis".

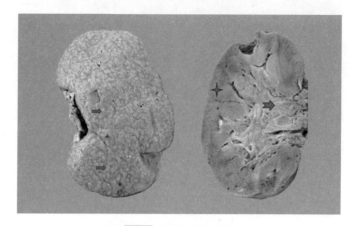

图 10-03　慢性肾小球肾炎

Fig. 10-03　Chronic glomerulonephritis

思考题：颗粒状的表面是如何形成的？

Question：How is the granular surface formed?

（二）肾盂肾炎 Pyelonephritis

慢性肾盂肾炎（图 10-04）：肾体积略变小，表面高低不平，有多处大小不一的凹陷疤痕。有的疤痕处（➡）残留有粘连的包膜，肾盂黏膜粗糙（★）。

Chronic pyelonephritis （Fig. 10-04）：The kidney volume is slightly smaller with uneven surface. There are many depressed scars of different sizes. Some of the scars（➡）have adhesive capsules，and the renal pelvis mucosa is rough（★）.

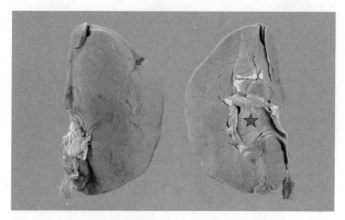

图 10-04　慢性肾盂肾炎

Fig. 10-04　Chronic pyelonephritis

（三）肿瘤 Tumors

（1）肾细胞癌（图 10-05）：正常肾组织（▲）被破坏，大部分肾组织被肿瘤（★）所替代。切面可见瘤组织呈灰白、灰黄色，有的伴大块棕褐色出血坏死区。

Renal cellular carcinoma（Fig. 10-05）：The normal part of the kidney（▲）is destroyed and replaced by the tumor（★）. The cut surface is grayish gray and grayish yellow, and some are accompanied by large brown hemorrhagic necrotic area.

（2）膀胱尿路上皮乳头状癌（图 10-06）：膀胱壁已被剪开，黏膜面有菜花状或乳头状肿瘤，基底部宽窄不一。

Urothelial papillocarcionoma of the urinary bladder（Fig. 10-06）：The urinary bladder wall has been cut, and the mucosal surface has cauliflower-like or papillary tumors, and the base is wide or narrow.

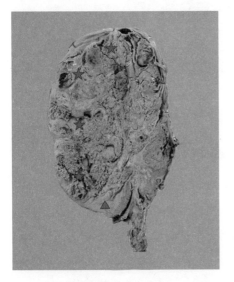

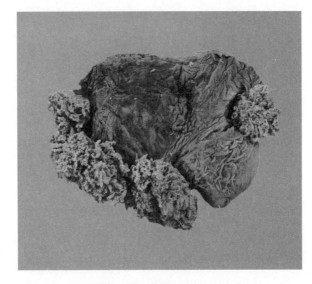

图 10-05　肾细胞癌

Fig. 10-05　Renal celluar carcinoma

图 10-06　膀胱尿路上皮乳头状癌

Fig. 10-06　Urothelial papillocarcionoma of the urinary bladder

（3）肾盂尿路上皮乳头状癌：请见第五章图 5-27 相关描述。

Urothelial papillocarcionoma of the pelvis：See Fig. 5-27 in Chapter 5.

三、组织切片观察 Observation of tissue slides

（1）急性弥漫增生性肾小球肾炎（图 10-07）：肾小球（★）体积增大，细胞数目明显增多，其中内皮细胞、球内系膜细胞增生及中性粒细胞浸润（图 10-07a）；部分肾小球毛细血管正常结构消失，发生纤维素样坏死，红染（图 10-07b），无结构状（➡）；肾小管上皮细胞混浊肿胀,腔内有红染蛋白性物质,即透明管型(▲);部分肾小管腔内可见大量红细胞,即红细胞管型(◥)。

Acute proliferative glomerulonephritis(Fig. 10-07): The glomerular (★) volume increased with significant number of cells, including endothelial cells, intracellular mesangial cells and neutrophil infiltration(Fig. 10-07a). Some of the normal structure of glomerular capillaries disappear, and undergo cellulose-like necrosis with red staining(Fig. 10-07b) and no structure (➡). Renal tubular epithelial cells showed turbid swelling, with red stained protein in the cavity, which is transparent cast (▲). A large number of red blood cells, which are red blood cell casts (◥) can be seen in some renal tubules.

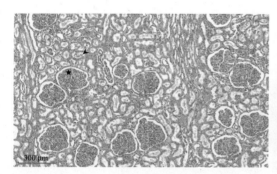 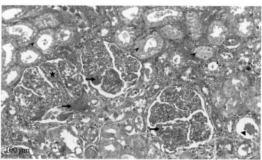

a. 低倍镜 lower magnification   b. 高倍镜 higher magnification

图 10-07　急性弥漫增生性肾小球肾炎

Fig. 10-07　Acute diffuse proliferative glomerulonephritis

（2）快速进行性肾小球肾炎（图 10-08）：肾小球囊壁层上皮细胞增生显著,围绕肾毛细血管丛形成环状体结构(★),少数呈半月形的新月体结构;肾小管近曲小管上皮细胞扁平,管腔扩大,腔内有蛋白管型(▲)、颗粒管型、细胞管型;伴有少量灶性淋巴细胞、单核细胞浸润。

Rapidly progressive glomerulonephritis(Fig. 10-08): The glomerular capsule wall epithelial cells proliferate significantly, forming a ring-shaped structure around the renal capillary plexus (★) or less frequently crescentic structures. Renal tubular proximal convoluted tubule epithelial cells are flat, lumens are enlarged, and there are protein casts (▲), granular casts, cellular casts; accompanied by a small amount of focal lymphocytes, mononuclear cell's infiltration.

（3）慢性肾小球肾炎（图 10-09）：大量肾小球纤维化及玻璃样变(★),相应的肾小管萎缩甚至消失,导致玻璃样变肾小球相互靠近(肾小球集中现象);少量肾小球代偿性肥大,球囊体积增大,相应周围所属肾小管管腔扩张(▲),肾小管内可见蛋白管型;肾间质纤维化伴有慢性炎细胞浸润,小动脉管壁内膜下纤维组织增生,管壁增厚,管腔狭窄(◥)。

Chronic glomerulonephritis(Fig. 10-09): A large number of glomeruli showed fibrosis and hyaline degeneration (★). The corresponding tubules undergo atrophy, or even disappear, leading to the hyalinized glomeruli close to each other (glomeruli concentration phenomenon). A small amount of glomeruli are compensatory hypertrophy, with increased volume, and the corresponding surrounding renal tubuls expand (▲). The protein casts are seen in renal tubular. Renal interstitium undergoes fibrosis, accompanied by chronic inflammatory cell infiltration. Small arterial wall sees subendocardial fibrous tissue hyperplasia, with thickened wall and narrow lumen (➤).

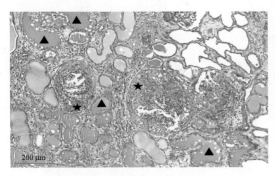

图 10-08　快速进行性肾小球肾炎
Fig. 10-08　Rapidly progressive glomerulonephritis

图 10-09　慢性肾小球肾炎
Fig. 10-09　Chronic glomerulonephritis

（4）急性肾盂肾炎（图 10-10）：以肾髓质病变为主（图 10-10a）者，间质内有大量中性粒细胞浸泡，有的形成小脓肿（★），部分肾小管管腔内亦有中性粒细胞，有的肾小管上皮脱落，肾小球病变轻微；以肾皮质病变为主（图 10-10b）者，可见散在多发性小脓肿形成（★），肾小管内有大量中性粒细胞，即白细胞管型（➤）。

Acute pyelonephritis（Fig. 10-10）：If it mainly involved the renal medullary (Fig. 10-10a), a large number of neutrophils are seen in the interstitial, and some form a small abscess (★). Some of the renal tubules also see neutrophils, and some tubular epithelial shed, with mild glomerular lesion. If it mainly involved the renal cortex (Fig. 10-10b), multiple scattered small abscess formed (★). A large number of neutrophils present in the renal tubules, namely white blood cell cast (➤).

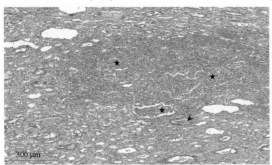

a. 肾髓质病变 renal medullary lesions

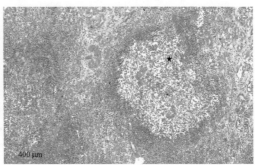

b. 肾皮质病变 renal cortical lesions

图 10-10　急性肾盂肾炎
Fig. 10-10　Acute pyelonephritis

（5）膀胱尿路上皮乳头状癌（图 10-11）：膀胱黏膜可见乳头状结构（★），分支较多且不规则；乳头中央为纤维血管轴心（➡），表面被覆 7～8 层甚至 10 多层的细胞，细胞呈梭形及椭圆形，部分有异型性，可见核分裂。

Urothelial papillocarcionoma of the urinary bladder（Fig. 10-11）：The bladder mucosa sees a papillary structure（★）with many branches and irregularities. The center of papilli is the fibro vascular core（➡），and the surface is covered with 7 – 8 to 10 layers of cells. The cells are fusiform and elliptical, and some showed atypia and mitotic image.

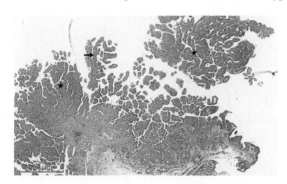 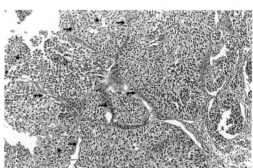

低倍镜 lower magnification　　　　　　高倍镜 higher magnification

图 10-11　膀胱尿路上皮乳头状癌

Fig. 10-11　Urothelium cell papillocarcionoma of the urinary bladder

四、　病例讨论 Case discussion

患儿，男，8 岁，因"眼睑水肿、尿少 2 天"入院。

患儿 1 周前曾发生上呼吸道感染。

体格检查：眼睑浮肿，咽红肿，心肺（－），血压 126/91mmHg。

实验室检查：尿常规检查显示红细胞（＋＋），尿蛋白（＋＋），红细胞管型每个高倍视野下 0～3 个;24 h 尿量 350 mL，尿素氮 11.4 mmol/L，血肌酐 170 μmol/L。B 超检查显示双肾对称性增大。

The child, male, 8 years old, was admitted to hospital due to edema of the eyelids and oliguria for 2 days.

Upper respiratory tract infection occurred 1 week ago.

Physical examination：eyelid edema, pharyngeal redness, heart and lung（－），blood pressure 126/91 mmHg.

Laboratory examination：urine routine, red blood cells（＋＋），urine protein（＋＋），red blood cell tube type 0 –3/HP; 24 h urine volume 350 mL, urea nitrogen 11.4 mmol/L, serum creatinine 170μmol/L. B-ultrasound：increased symmetry of the kidneys.

分析题 Questions

（1）请做出诊断并描述诊断依据。

Please make a diagnosis and describe the basis of diagnosis.

（2）请描述该患者的临床病理联系。

Please describe the patient's clinical pathology.

五、 思考题 Questions

（1）急性肾小球肾炎患者出现血尿、蛋白尿和高血压的病理基础是什么？

What is the pathological basis of hematuria, proteinuria and hypertension in patients with acute glomerulonephritis?

（2）慢性肾小球肾炎的主要病理变化有哪些？试应用病理学知识解释该病患者的高血压、氮质血症和代谢性酸中毒等症状。

What are the main pathological changes of chronic glomerulonephritis? Apply pathological knowledge to explain the symptoms of hypertension, azotemia and metabolic acidosis in patients with this disease.

（3）急性肾小球肾炎和肾盂肾炎的发病机制、病理变化及主要临床表现有何不同？

What is the difference in the pathogenesis, pathological changes and main clinical manifestations of acute glomerulonephritis and pyelonephritis?

（4）膀胱癌的病理类型和特点是什么？

What are the pathological types and characteristics of urinary bladder cancer?

（5）名词解释：肾病综合征、Goodpasture 综合征、颗粒性固缩肾、新月体。

Terms explanation：nephrotic syndrome, Goodpasture syndrome, granular pyknosis, crescent.

编写 Written by：刘瑶 Liu Yao

中文审校 Chinese proofreader：邓敏 Deng Min

英文审校 English proofreader：刘瑶 Liu Yao

一、 教学目的 Teaching objectives

（1）掌握子宫颈癌与乳腺癌的病变特点。

Master the characteristics of the cervical cancer and the breast cancer.

（2）熟悉葡萄胎、绒毛膜上皮癌的病变特点。

Be familiar with the characteristics of hydatidiform mole and choriocarcinoma.

（3）了解前列腺肥大和阴茎癌的病变特点。

Understand the characteristics of the benign prostate hyperplasia and the penile cancer.

二、 大体标本观察 Observation of gross specimens

（一）子宫颈病变 Diseases of cervix

（1）子宫颈癌（溃疡型）（图 11-01）：宫颈处（➡）表面组织溃烂，向下凹陷。

Cervical carcinoma（ulcerative type）（Fig. 11-01）: The surface of the cervix（➡）is ulcerated and sagged downward.

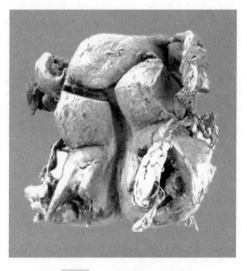

图 11-01　子宫颈癌（溃疡型）

Fig. 11-01　Cervical carcinoma（ulcerative type）

（2）子宫颈癌（外生菜花型）（图 11-02）：宫腔及宫颈已被剪开,灰白色的癌组织向表面生长,并呈菜花状（➡）。

Cervical carcinoma（exogenous cauliflower type）（Fig. 11-02）：The uterine cavity and the cervix have been cut. The grayish white cancer tissue grows to the surface and is cauliflower-like（➡）.

（3）子宫颈癌（内生浸润型）（图 11-03）：灰白色癌组织呈弥漫性浸润宫颈,并已向颈管浸润（➡）。

Cervical carcinoma（internal infiltrative type）（Fig. 11-03）：The gray-white cancer tissue infiltrated diffusely in the cervix, as well as into the cervical canal（➡）.

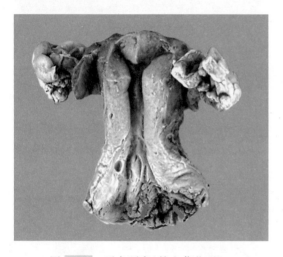 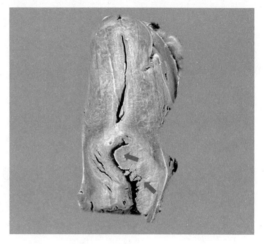

图 11-02 子宫颈癌（外生菜花型）　　　图 11-03 子宫颈癌（内生浸润型）
Fig. 11-02 Cervical carcinoma（exogenous cauliflower type）　　　Fig. 11-03 Cervical carcinoma（internal infiltrative type）

（二）滋养层细胞病变 Diseases of trophoblast

（1）葡萄胎（图 11-04）：子宫腔内被半透明的水泡状物（➡）填满。

Hydatidiform mole（Fig. 11-04）：The uterine cavity is filled with translucent bubbles（➡）.

（2）侵蚀性葡萄胎（图 11-05）：子宫腔内可见半透明的水泡状物,部分水泡状物浸润子宫壁（➡）。

Invasive mole（Fig. 11-05）：The translucent bubbles are found in the uterine cavity, and some of them infiltrated into the uterine wall（➡）.

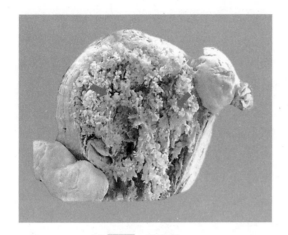

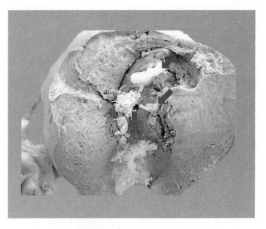

图 11-04 葡萄胎

Fig. 11-04 Hydatidiform mole

图 11-05 侵蚀性葡萄胎

Fig. 11-05 Invasive mole

（3）绒毛膜癌（图 11-06）：子宫腔壁上有结节状癌组织，呈灰白色和暗褐色。癌组织突向宫腔（➡），底部向宫壁深层浸润，部分癌组织已经穿透子宫全层（➡）。

Choriocarcinoma（Fig. 11-06）：Nodular carcinoma on the wall of the uterus is grayish and dark-brown. The cancer tissue protrudes into the uterine cavity（➡）, and the bottom penetrates deep into the uterine wall, and some have penetrated the whole layers（➡）

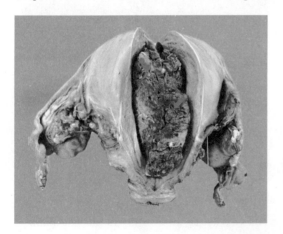

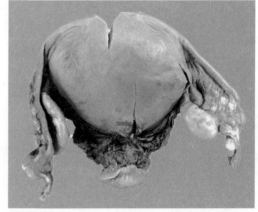

图 11-06 绒毛膜癌

Fig. 11-06 Choriocarcinoma

（4）绒毛膜癌肝脏转移（图 11-07）：肝脏切面上可见多个癌结节（★），大部分结节靠近肝脏被膜。在结节中心部可见灰黄色坏死区域；在结节边缘处可见明显呈黑色的出血区域。

Metastatic choriocarcinoma of the liver（Fig. 11-07）：Multiple nodular cancer lesions（★）are found on the liver section, and most of the nodules are close to the liver capsule. The gray-yellow necrotic area is found in the center of the nodule and there is a black bleeding area at the edge of the nodule.

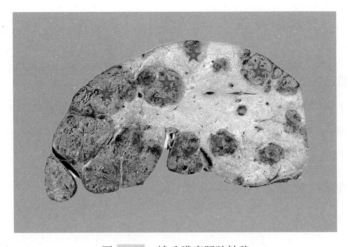

图 11-07　绒毛膜癌肝脏转移

Fig. 11-07　Metastatic choriocarcinoma of the liver

（三）卵巢肿瘤 Tumors of the ovarium

（1）卵巢黏液性囊腺瘤（图 11-08）：肿瘤切面可见多个囊腔,囊腔内可见胶冻状物
（➡）。

Ovarian mucinous cystadenoma（Fig. 11-08）：Multiple cystic cavities can be found on the
tumor section, and jelly-like substance（➡）can be found in the cystic cavities.

（2）卵巢成熟畸胎瘤（图 11-09）：肿瘤呈囊状。囊腔内可见黑色毛发和黄色脂肪。

Ovarian mature teratoma（Fig. 11-09）：The tumor is cystic. Black hair and yellow fat are
found in the cyst.

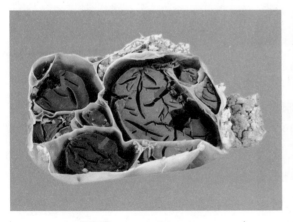

图 11-08　卵巢黏液性囊腺瘤

Fig. 11-08　Ovarian mucinous cystadenoma

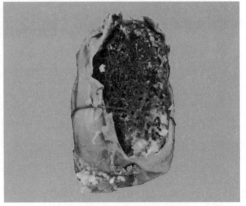

图 11-09　卵巢成熟畸胎瘤

Fig. 11-09　Ovarian mature teratoma

（四）乳腺肿瘤 Tumors of the breast

乳腺癌（图 11-10）：此标本显示乳腺的切面，切面上可见明显的灰白色癌组织（▲），癌组织浸润入脂肪组织中；并且可见乳头内陷（➡）。

Carcinoma of the breast（Fig. 11-10）：This specimen shows the cut surface of breast. The obvious grayish white cancer tissue（▲）is found and the cancer tissue infiltrates into the adipose tissue. Also, the nipple retraction（➡）can be found.

（五）男性生殖系统疾病 Diseases of the male genital system

（1）睾丸精原细胞瘤（图 11-11）：睾丸增大，白膜未被破坏。切面可见睾丸被实体性肿瘤取代，呈灰白色，质地细腻。

Seminoma of the testis（Fig. 11-11）：The testicle become big and the tunica albuginea is not destroyed. On the cut surface, the testicle is replaced by solid tumors, which are grayish white and fine in texture.

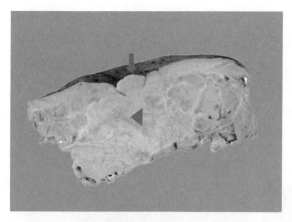
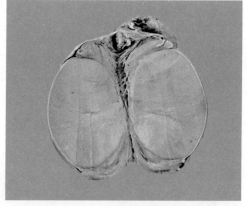

图 11-10 乳腺癌 | 图 11-11 睾丸精原细胞瘤
Fig. 11-10 Carcinoma of the breast | Fig. 11-11 Seminoma of the testis

（2）前列腺增生症（图 11-12）：前列腺包膜完整，切面呈结节状，黄白色。

Benign prostatic hyperplasia（Fig. 11-12）：The prostate capsule is intact; the section is nodular, shows yellow-white.

（3）阴茎鳞癌（图 11-13）：在阴茎头部可见菜花状肿块（➡）。

Squamous cell carcinoma of the penis（Fig. 11-13）：A cauliflower-like mass（➡）can be found on the head of the penis.

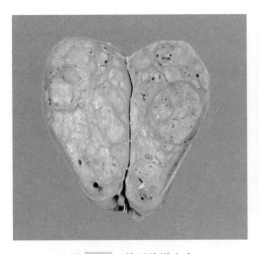
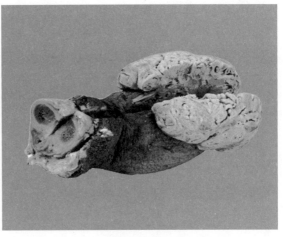

图 11-12　前列腺增生症
Fig. 11-12　Benign prostatic hyperplasia

图 11-13　阴茎鳞癌
Fig. 11-13　Squamous cell carcinoma of the penis

三、组织切片观察 Observation of tissue slides

（1）葡萄胎（图11-14）：绒毛间质高度水肿（★），导致绒毛肿大；绒毛间质内未见血管或血管内无红细胞；绒毛表面的滋养叶细胞增生显著。增生的细胞包括内层的细胞滋养层细胞（➤）及外层的合体滋养层细胞（➡）。

Hydatidiform mole（Fig. 11-14）：The interstitial edema（★）results in swollen villi. There are no blood vessels or no red blood cells in the villi. The trophoblastic proliferation is found on the surface of villi. Proliferating cells include inner cytotrophoblasts（➤）and outer syncytiotrophoblasts（➡）.

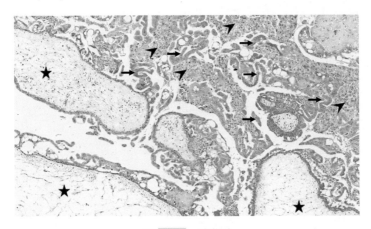

图 11-14　葡萄胎
Fig. 11-14　Hydatidiform mole

（2）绒毛膜癌（图 11-15）：子宫壁肌层内有绒癌组织（★）浸润，不形成绒毛结构。浸润的癌细胞包括两种数量不等的恶性滋养叶细胞：细胞滋养层样癌细胞（◥）及合体滋养层细胞样癌细胞（➡）。癌细胞间无血管及间质。肿瘤细胞直接侵入子宫肌内，有大片出血坏死（▲）。

Choriocarcinoma（Fig. 11-15）：Choriocarcinoma tissue（★）is in the uterine wall muscle layer, it does not form a villus structure. The infiltrating cancer cells include two kinds of malignant trophoblast cells：Cytotrophoblast-like cancer cells（◥）and syncytiotrophoblast-like cancer cells（➡）. There are no blood vessels and interstitial cells among the cancer cells. The cancer cells invade into the uterine muscle. There are large pieces of hemorrhagic necrosis（▲）.

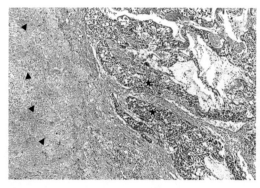 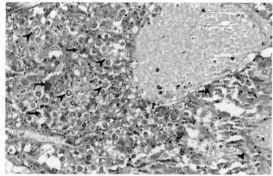

低倍镜 lower magnification　　　　高倍镜 higher magnification

图 11-15　绒毛膜癌
Fig. 11-15　Choriocarcinoma

（3）前列腺增生（图 11-16）：前列腺腺体显著增生（★），腺体上皮数目增多，排列紧密，有的呈乳头状突出于腔内，有的呈囊状扩张，其上皮已变成扁平状；腺腔内可见红染的分泌物（混杂有脱落上皮及白细胞），有的凝集成同心圆状（前列腺小体）（▲）；腺体之间的平滑肌（◥）及结缔组织也增生（➡）。

Benign prostatic hyperplasia（Fig. 11-16）：Proliferative prostate get glandular hyperplasia（★）. Glandular epithelial increased, closely arranged, some are papillary protruding to the cavity, and some are cystic dilated. The epithelium has become flat. The red stained secretions（mixed with epithelial and white blood cells）are visible in the glandular cavity, and some are concentric（corpora amylacea）（▲）. Smooth muscles between the glands（◥）and connective tissues also proliferate（➡）.

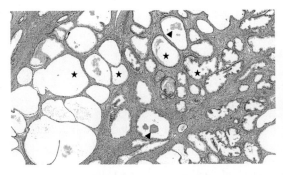 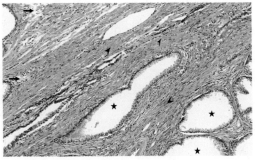

低倍镜 lower magnification　　　　　　　高倍镜 higher magnification

图 11-16　前列腺增生

Fig. 11-16　Benign hyperplasia of the prostate

（4）乳腺浸润性导管癌（图 11-17）：正常乳腺组织全被癌组织取代,部分癌细胞主要局限于导管内,排列成各种不规则的巢状(★)。癌细胞呈实性排列,中央可见坏死(◥);部分为条索状(➡),偶尔形成腺样结构。癌巢间有纤维组织及淋巴细胞浸润(▲)。

Invasive ductal carcinoma of the breast (Fig. 11-17): Normal breast tissues are completely replaced by cancer tissues, and some cancer cells are mainly confined to the duct, arranged in various irregular nests(★). The cancer cells are arranged in a solid mass with necrosis (◥) in the center; other cancer cells are arranged in the cords (➡), adenoid structures are occasionally formed. The fibrous tissue and lymphocyte infiltration (▲) are in the interstitial spaces of the cancer.

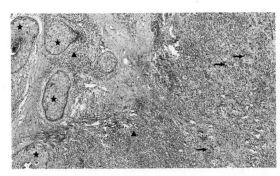 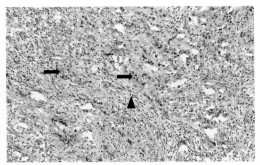

低倍镜 lower magnification　　　　　　　高倍镜 higher magnification

图 11-17　乳腺浸润性导管癌

Fig. 11-17　Invasive ductal carcinoma of the breast

四、　病例讨论 Case discussion

患者,女,29 岁。因发现盆腔肿块予以手术治疗。

手术中医生发现患者右侧卵巢肿块，考虑是卵巢肿瘤。

病理学标本检查：肿瘤为灰白和灰红色组织，有大小不等的囊腔，囊腔内可见毛发、油脂、骨及软骨。显微镜下可见肿瘤分化成熟的部分有鳞状上皮、各种腺上皮、骨及软骨等，分化不成熟的组织有不成熟的间叶组织及大量原始神经组织。

Patient, female, 29 years old, underwent surgery due to a pelvic mass.

The right ovarian mass was found during surgery and the doctor considered ovarian tumors.

Pathological specimen examination: The tumor is grayish and gray-red tissue, in which there are cysts of different sizes, in which hair, oil, bone and cartilage are found. Microscopically, the tumor differentiated mature parts include squamous epithelium, various glandular epithelium, bone and cartilage. The immature tissues include immature mesenchymal tissue and a large number of primitive neural tissues.

思考题 Questions

（1）根据病例资料做出病理诊断，并写出理由。

Make a pathological diagnosis based on the case data and write the reasons.

（2）手术标本包含有哪些胚层的成分？

What are the components of the germ layer in the surgical specimen?

五、 思考题 Questions

（1）宫颈癌的病理类型有哪些？其扩散途径如何？

What are the pathological types of cervical cancer and how do they spread?

（2）简述乳腺癌的组织学类型及扩散方式。

Briefly describe the histological type and spread of the breast cancer.

（3）请列举卵巢常见肿瘤的病变特点及临床表现。

Please list the pathological features and clinical manifestations of common ovarian tumors.

（4）请写出葡萄胎、恶性葡萄胎和绒毛膜上皮癌的病理改变和临床特征的异同点。

Please write out the similarities and differences of pathological changes and clinical features between hydatidiform mole, malignant mole and chorionic epithelial cancer.

编写 Written by：董亮 Dong Liang

中文审校 Chinese proofreader：邓敏 Deng Min

英文审校 English proofreader：刘瑶 Liu Yao

第十二章　内分泌系统（甲状腺）疾病

Chapter 12　Diseases of the Endocrine System (Thyroid)

一、　教学目的 Teaching objectives

（1）掌握非毒性和毒性甲状腺肿的基本病理变化及其与临床的联系。

Master the morphological changes and clinical features of nontoxic and toxic goiter.

（2）熟悉甲状腺常见肿瘤的类型和形态特点。

Be familiar with the classification and the morphology of the thyroid neoplasms.

二、　大体标本观察 Observation of gross specimens

（一）甲状腺肿 Enlargement of the thyroid (goiter)

（1）弥漫性胶性甲状腺肿（图 12-01）：甲状腺弥漫性均匀性肿大，表面光滑，无结节（图 12-01a），切面较均匀，富有棕红色半透明胶质。有的标本切面已有少数结节（★）形成（图 12-01b）（向结节性甲状腺肿发展）。

Diffuse colloid goiter (Fig. 12-01): The thyroid is enlarged diffusely, with a smooth surface (Fig. 12-01a) and a uniform cut surface. The hyperplastic follicles contain abundant reddish-brown colloid within the lumina. Some of these specimens already have nodule formation (Fig. 12-01b ★), which indicates the progression of the disease to multinodular goiter.

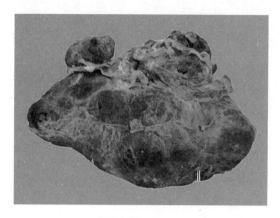
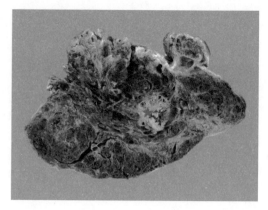

a. 表面光滑 smooth surface　　　　　b. 切面有少数结节形成 nodule formation

图 12-01　弥漫性胶性甲状腺肿

Fig. 12-01　Diffuse colloid goiter

（2）结节性甲状腺肿（图 12-02）：甲状腺肿大，但不均匀，表面呈结节状，切面可见甲状腺内布满大小不等的结节（★）。多数结节境界不清，或者局部境界清楚，有纤维性间隔（➡），但尚未形成完整的纤维性包膜。有的结节有囊性变。

Multinodular goiter（Fig. 12-02）：The thyroid gland is enlarged asymmetrically with a coarse surface. Multiple nodules（★）with varying sizes are observed on the cut surface. Most nodules do not have complete capsules, only focal fibrinous septum is found（➡）. A few nodules have complete fibrinous capsule, which leads to fibrocystic changes of nodules.

（3）毒性甲状腺肿（图 12-03）：甲状腺肿大，滤泡扩大，充满淡黄色的半透明胶质。间质结缔组织稍有增加。

Toxic goiter（Fig. 12-03）：The thyroid gland is enlarged with hyperplastic follicles which contain abundant transparent yellow colloid. Moderate interstitial fibrosis can take place.

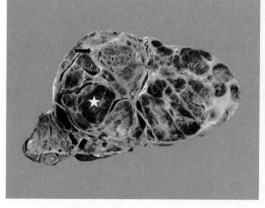
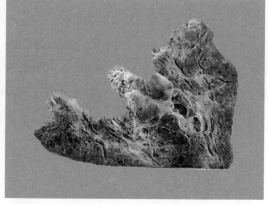

图 12-02　结节性甲状腺肿　　　　　　图 12-03　毒性甲状腺肿

Fig. 12-02　Multinodular goiter　　　　Fig. 12-03　Toxic goiter

（二）甲状腺肿瘤 The thyroid neoplasms

（1）甲状腺腺瘤（图12-04）：球状团块，有包膜（➡）。瘤块切面呈棕褐色和灰红色，有出血（★）。

The thyroid adenoma（Fig. 12-04）: Two spheroidal neoplasms with capsules（➡）. The cut surface of neoplasms have brown or dark brown appearance, companied by hemorrhage（★） inside the lesion.

（2）甲状腺乳头状癌（图12-05）：肿块不规则，切面可见乳头状白色实体物（➡），境界不清。

The thyroid papillary carcinoma（Fig. 12-05）: These neoplasms are multifocal. In this cross-section, white papillary excrescences（➡） without a clear boarder are present.

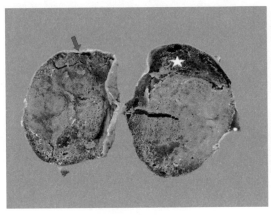

图 12-04　甲状腺腺瘤
Fig. 12-04　Thyroid adenoma

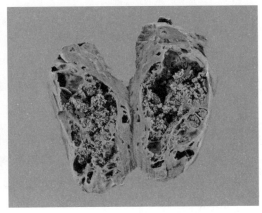

图 12-05　甲状腺乳头状癌
Fig. 12-05　Thyroid papillary carcinoma

三、组织切片观察 Observation of tissue slides

（1）弥漫性胶性甲状腺肿（图12-06）：甲状腺滤泡由于腔内胶质（★）的贮积而高度扩张，腺腔大小不一，上皮变低立方或扁平（➡），偶可见残留的增生的小乳头（▲）。

Diffuse colloid goiter（Fig. 12-06）: Follicles of thyroid are enlarged dramatically because of the storage of abundant colloid（★）. The enlarged follicles are in different sizes. Epithelium has a columnar and flattened appearance（➡）. Sometimes remaining small papillary patterns can be observed（▲）.

（2）毒性甲状腺肿（图12-07）：甲状腺滤泡增多，滤泡大小不一，以小滤泡为主（★），滤泡上皮多数呈立方或低柱状，少数为乳头状增生（◀）；滤泡腔内胶质稀少，靠近滤泡上皮的胶质内出现排列成行的空泡（吸收空泡）（➡）；间质中可见到淋巴细胞浸润（▲）。

Toxic goiter (Fig. 12-07): In this section, more follicles with variable sizes are observed. Majority of these follicles are small follicles (★), which flattened and columnar epithelial cells and sometimes papillation (✔) are observed. There are less colloid inside follicles, therefore small and clear vacuoles (absorbing vacuoles) (➡) are present around the epithelium. Interstitial lymphocyte infiltration (▲) is observed.

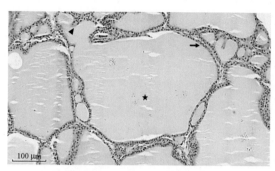

图 12-06　弥漫性胶性甲状腺肿
Fig. 12-06　Diffuse colloid goiter

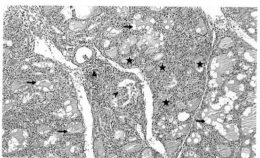

图 12-07　毒性甲状腺肿
Fig. 12-07　Toxic goiter

四、　病例讨论 Case discussion

患者,女,28 岁,因心悸、怕热、多汗、食欲亢进、体重减轻来医院诊治。

体格检查:体温 37 ℃,脉率 99 次/分,眼球突出,双侧甲状腺弥漫性、对称性肿大。基础代谢率明显升高。

实验室检查:T_3、T_4 水平升高,甲状腺摄^{131}I 率增高。入院后行甲状腺次全切除术。

病理检查:肉眼可见甲状腺弥漫性肿大,表面光滑。切面质实,色灰红。镜下可见甲状腺滤泡弥漫性增生,上皮细胞呈柱状,并形成乳状结构突向滤泡腔。滤泡腔较小,腔内胶质少而稀薄,靠近上边缘有成排的吸收空泡。间质充血,有大量淋巴细胞浸润并有淋巴滤泡形成。

A 28-year old female, had palpitations, swelling, excessive appetite and obvious weight-loss.

Physical examination: Temperature 37℃, pulse 99 times per minute, exophthalmos, diffuse enlargement of bilateral thyroids, and high basal metabolic rate.

Laboratory examination: Elevated T_3, T_4 levels and iodine uptake rate of thyroid were detected. Subtotal thyroidectomy was carried out for the patient.

Pathological examination: Macroscopically, thyroids were diffusely enlarged and the surface was glossy, while the cut surface of specimen had a hard and dark-red appearance. Microscopically, there was diffuse hyperplasia of thyroid follicles, surrounded by columnar epithelial cells, which formed papilla towards the lumen of follicles. The follicles are reduced in size and had much less colloid with a watery appearance. Absorbing vacuoles were present in the periphery of follicles. Hyperemia, lymphocyte infiltration and formation of lymphoid follicles were found in the interstitium.

问题 Questions

（1）你的病理诊断是什么？请提供诊断依据。

What is your diagnosis? Please give evidences for your diagnosis.

（2）请根据病理变化分析临床病理联系。

Please explain the clinical symptoms according to the pathological change of disease.

（3）除本例外，请列出还有哪些疾病能导致甲状腺弥漫性肿大。

Please give other examples of disease which can lead to the enlargement of the thyroid.

五、　思考题 Questions

（1）地方性甲状腺肿与甲亢在发病机制、病理变化和预后上有哪些不同？

Compare endemic goiter and hyperthyroidism according to the pathogenesis, pathological changes and clinical prognosis.

（2）总结结节性甲状腺肿和甲状腺腺瘤的区别。

Summarize the difference between the nodular goiter and the thyroid adenoma.

（3）甲状腺癌有哪些类型？病理变化是什么？

What are the classification and pathological changes of the thyroid adenocarcinoma?

4. 名词解释：非毒性甲状腺肿、克汀病、APUD 瘤。

Please explain: nontoxic goiter, cretinism and apudoma.

编写 Written by：万珊 Wan Shan

中文审校 Chinese proofreader：邓敏 Deng Min

英文审校 English proofreader：刘瑶 Liu Yao

13

第十三章 神经系统疾病

Chapter 13 Diseases of the Nervous System

一、教学目的 Teaching objectives

（1）掌握流行性脑脊髓膜炎的病理特点。

Master the morphologic changes of the epidemic meningitis.

（2）掌握乙型脑炎的病理特点。

Master the morphologic changes of the encephalitis B.

二、大体标本观察 Observation of gross specimens

（一）炎症性病变 Inflammatory lesions

（1）流行性脑脊髓膜炎（图13-01）：脑膜血管充血（➡），蛛网膜下腔有较多混浊不清的灰黄色脓性渗出物积聚（★）。

Epidemic cerebrospinal meningitis （Fig. 13-01）：Arachnoid membrane become cloudy and meningeal vessels are remarkably congested （➡）. The subarachnoid space contains grey yellow cloudy suppurative exudation（★）.

（2）暴发型脑膜炎球菌性败血症——肾上腺出血（图13-02）：两侧肾上腺广泛出血（★）。

Fulminant meningococcemia—hemorrhage of the adrenal gland （Fig. 13-02）：The adrenal gland is hemorrhagic（★）.

三、组织切片观察 Observation of tissue slides

（一）炎症性病变 Inflammatory lesions

（1）流行性脑脊髓膜炎（图13-03）：蛛网膜下腔高度扩大，内有大量中性粒细胞及一些单核细胞浸润（➡），并有较多纤维素渗出，

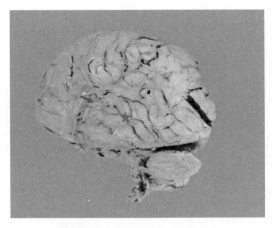

图 13-01　流行性脑脊髓膜炎

Fig. 13-01　Epidemic cerebrospinal meningitis

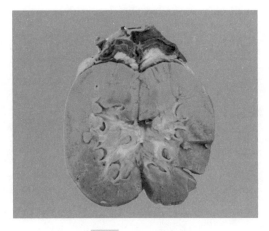

图 13-02　肾上腺出血

Fig. 13-02　Hemorrhage of the adrenal gland

血管扩张充血（✦）。脑实质（★）病变不明显。

Epidemic cerebrospinal meningitis (Fig. 13-03)：The subarachnoid space is highly enlarged, with a large number of neutrophils and some mononuclear cells' infiltration （➡）, and much fibrous exudation, vasodilatation and hyperemia （✦）. Brain parenchymal （★） lesions are not obvious.

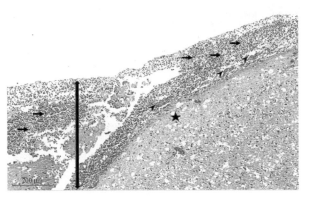

图 13-03　流行性脑脊髓膜炎

Fig. 13-03　Epidemic cerebrospinal meningitis

（2）乙型脑炎（图 13-04）：脑血管周围间隙扩张，其中有多量淋巴细胞浸润形成淋巴细胞套（★）。脑实质中有多数散在分布的染色浅而结构疏松的软化灶，该处神经元、胶质细胞均消失，仅残留网状支架，即筛状软化灶（▲）。在变性的神经元周围，有数个少突胶质细胞围绕，形成神经细胞卫星现象（➡）。小胶质细胞吞噬变性坏死的神经元，称为噬神经现象。胶质细胞轻度弥漫增生，少数区域形成小团块，称为胶质细胞小结。

Encephalitis B （Fig. 13-04）：The perivascular space is dilated, and a large number of lymphocytes infiltrate to form a lymphocyte sheath （★）. There are mostly scattered pale-stained and loosely-structured softening lesions in the brain parenchyma. The neurons and glial cells disappeared, leaving only the reticular scaffold, i. e. the sieve-like softening lesion （▲）. Around the degenerated neurons, several oligodendrocytes surround each other to form a neuronal satellite （➡）. Microglia phagocytose degeneration and necrosis of neurons, called neuronophagia. Glial cells are slightly diffuse and proliferate, and a small number of areas form small clumps, called glial cell nodules.

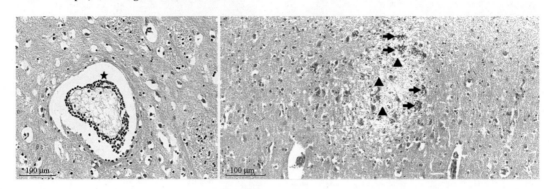

图 13-04　乙型脑炎

Fig. 13-04　Encephalitis B

四、思考题 Questions

（1）流行性脑脊髓膜炎的病变特点及其临床病理联系有哪些？

What are the characteristics of pathological changes in epidemic cerebrospinal meningitis and its clinical pathological relationship?

（2）乙型脑炎的病变特点有哪些？

What are the basic pathological changes of encephalitis B?

（3）流行性脑脊髓膜炎与乙型脑炎有何不同？

What are the differences between epidemic cerebrospinal meningitis and encephalitis B?

（4）名词解释：红色神经元、噬神经细胞现象、Waterhous-Friedricsen 综合征、神经细胞卫星现象。

Definition：red neuron, neuronophagia, Waterhous-Friedricsen syndrome, satellitosis.

编写 Written by：谢芳 Xie Fang

中文审校 Chinese proofreader：邓敏 Deng Min

英文审校 English proofreader：刘瑶 Liu Yao

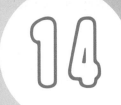

第十四章　感染性疾病

Chapter 14　Infectious Diseases

一、　教学目的 Teaching objectives

（1）掌握结核病的发病机制及转归,原发性与继发性肺结核病的病理变化及转归,常见肺外器官结核病的病理特点。

Master the pathogenesis and prognosis of tuberculosis, the pathological changes and prognosis of primary and secondary tuberculosis, and the pathological features of extrapulmonary tuberculosis.

（2）掌握伤寒、细菌性痢疾的病理变化。

Master the pathological changes of typhoid fever and bacillary dysentery.

（3）掌握血吸虫病的病理变化。

Master the pathological changes of schistosomiasis.

（4）熟悉阿米巴病的病理变化。

Be familiar with the pathological changes of amoebiasis.

（5）了解性传播疾病的主要病理变化。

Understand the pathological changes of sexually transmitted diseases.

二、　大体标本观察 Observation of gross specimens

（一）结核病概述 Overview of tuberculosis

（1）纤维包裹（肺结核球,图14-01）:肺切面上有一个圆球形结核病灶（结核球）,中央的干酪样坏死（★）被较厚的且已玻璃样变的纤维组织包裹（➡）。

Fibrous encapsulation (pulmonary tuberculoma, Fig. 14- 01）: A round lesion of tuberculosis (tuberculoma) is found on the cut surface, with caseous necrotic lesions (★) in the center and hyaline changes of thick connective tissue (➡) in the periphery.

（2）钙化（图 14-02）：肺部的结核病变已钙化，如石灰样小点（➡）。

Calcification（Fig. 14-02）：Calcification happens in the older lesions of tuberculosis，which appears as spots of lime（➡）.

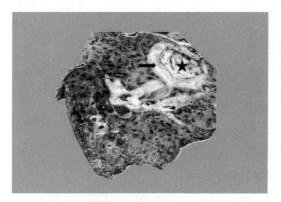
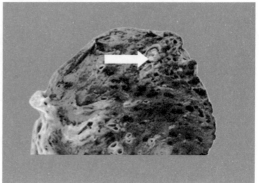

图 14-01　纤维包裹（肺结核球）

Fig. 14-01　Fibrous encapsulation

（pulmonary tuberculoma）

图 14-02　钙化

Fig. 14-02　Calcification

（3）自然管道播散及空洞形成 Nature canal dissemination and cavitation

① 急性空洞（图 14-03）：上叶有大片干酪样坏死及急性空洞（➡），下叶可见多数沿支气管散布的小的干酪样病灶（★）。

Acute cavitation（Fig. 14-03）：The upper lobes show massive areas of caseous necrosis companied by acute cavities formation（➡），while the lower lobes show small and disseminated caseous lesions lining around the bronchi（★）.

② 肾脏空洞（图 14-04）：肾脏有干酪样坏死灶及数个空洞（★），输尿管与膀胱也均可有结核病变。

Cavitation of kidney（Fig. 14-04）：This kidney has several lesions of caseous necrosis and cavities（★），which also happens in ureter and urinary bladder.

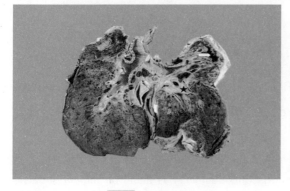
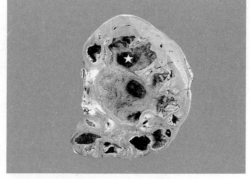

图 14-03　急性空洞

Fig. 14-03　Acute cavitation

图 14-04　肾脏空洞（肾结核病）

Fig. 14-04　Cavitation of kidney（tuberculosis of the kidney）

（4）淋巴道播散 Lymphatic dissemination

淋巴结结核（图 14-05）：标本为一组手术切除的颈部淋巴结，可见淋巴结明显增大（★），正常结构部分被破坏且被干酪样坏死物替代。

Tuberculosis of lymph nodes（Fig. 14-05）：This specimen is a group of cervical lymph nodes after surgical resection. Some lymph nodes are enlarged obviously（★）, in which the normal structure is replaced by caseous necrotic mass.

（5）血道播散 Hematogenous dissemination

粟粒性肺结核（图 14-06）：肺切面可见布满粟粒大的灰白、灰黄色结核病灶。

Miliary pulmonary tuberculosis（Fig. 14-06）：Note that the cut surface of the lung is full of grey-white lesions which are similar to miliaris in appearance.

思考题：请你补充一下结核病的转归还有哪些方面？

Question：What are the additional outcomes of tuberculosis according to the natural history of disease？

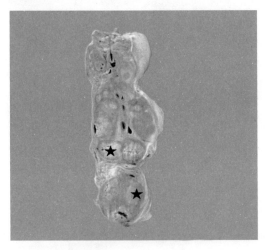
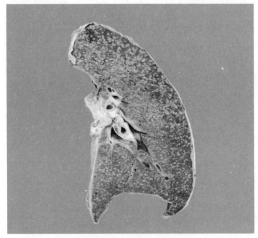

图 14-05　淋巴结结核

Fig. 14-05　Tuberculosis of lymph nodes

图 14-06　粟粒性肺结核

Fig. 14-06　Miliary pulmonary tuberculosis

（二）肺结核病 Tuberculosis

1. 原发性肺结核病及其病变进展 Primary tuberculosis and progression of disease

（1）原发性肺结核伴原发性空洞（图 14-07）：小儿肺脏标本。右肺中叶外侧近肺膜处可见一扩大的原发病灶，部分形成空洞，空洞约白果大小，内有干酪样坏死组织（★），肺门淋巴结肿大（➡），切面上亦可见干酪样坏死灶。

Primary pulmonary tuberculosis with primary cavitation（Fig. 14-07）：Lung specimen from a child. There is a primary lesion on the lateral side of mid lung field. Note that the enlarged primary lesion already has cavitation（★）, which looks like a ginkgo in size and has caseous necrosis in the center. There is obvious enlargement of hilar lymph nodes (➡), which is companied by caseous necrosis.

（2）原发性肺结核伴血源播散（图 14-08）：小儿肺脏标本。左肺下叶上部外侧近肺膜处可见一黄豆大原发病灶（★），肺门淋巴结肿大（➡），可见干酪样坏死。除上述病变外，还可见散在的粟粒大的灰黄色干酪样坏死灶（▲）。

Primary pulmonary tuberculosis with hematogenous dissemination （Fig. 14-08）：Lung specimen from a child. There is a subpleural primary lesion on the apical side of the inferior lobe, which appears like a soya bean in size （★）. There is obvious enlargement of hilar lymph nodes （➡） with caseous necrosis. In addition, there are multitude of miliary-looking caseous necrotic lesions scattered throughout the lung parenchyma （▲）.

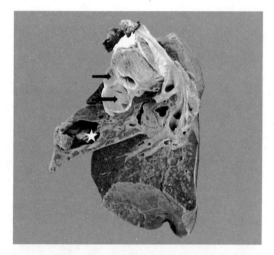 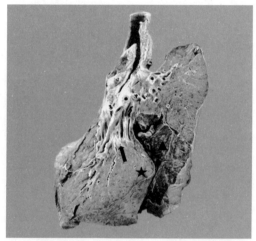

图 14-07　原发性肺结核伴原发性空洞
Fig. 14-07　Primary pulmonary tuberculosis with primary cavitation

图 14-08　原发性肺结核伴血源播散
Fig. 14-08　Primary pulmonary tuberculosis with hematogenous dissemination

（3）粟粒性肺结核（图 14-09）：肺组织中有散在的粟粒大的灰黄色干酪样坏死灶。

Miliary pulmonary tuberculosis （Fig. 14-09）：Small grey-yellow caseous necrotic lesions are scattered in the lung parenchyma.

2. 继发性肺结核病 Secondary pulmonary tuberculosis

（1）局灶型肺结核病伴钙化（图 14-10）：肺尖部有灶性结核病变（➡），边缘较整齐。

Focal pulmonary tuberculosis with calcification （Fig. 14-10）：There is a focal lesion on the apical side of the lung, with an orderly margin （➡）.

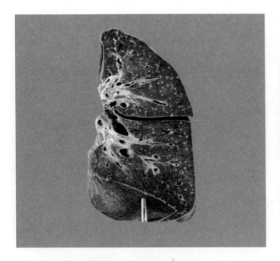

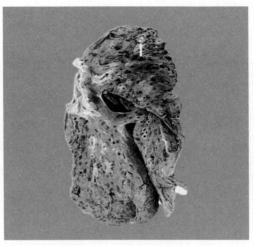

图 14-09 粟粒性肺结核

Fig. 14-09 Miliary pulmonary tuberculosis

图 14-10 局灶型肺结核病伴钙化

Fig. 14-10 Focal pulmonary tuberculosis
with calcification

（2）浸润型肺结核病（图 14-11）：肺部结核病灶与周围组织境界不清,病灶中央有干酪样坏死(➡)。有的标本病灶逐渐扩大,部分融合,附近尚可见许多粟粒大的支气管播散病灶。

Infiltrative pulmonary tuberculosis (Fig. 14-11): The pulmonary lesions do not have a clear boarder, with caseous necrosis in the center(➡). Adjacent lesions fused to a bigger one with the progression of lesions. Many small miliary-looking lesions are found infiltrating around the bronchi.

（3）浸润型肺结核病伴急性空洞（图 14-12）：肺切面上,上叶近肺尖部局灶肺组织发生干酪样坏死,部分坏死物经支气管排出后形成薄壁空洞(★),周围胸膜粗糙、增厚(▲),纤维组织增生;下叶有多数沿支气管分布的小的干酪样病灶(➡)。

Infiltrative pulmonary tuberculosis with acute cavitation (Fig. 14-12): On the cut surface of the lung, the upper lobe near the apex of lung showed caseous necrosis, When the necrotic mass is discarded through the bronchi, it leaves a cavity with a thin capsule at the primary site (★), the surrounding pleura of the cavity are rough, thickened (▲), and the fibrous tissue proliferated. Note that there are many small caseous granuloma lining around the bronchi (➡).

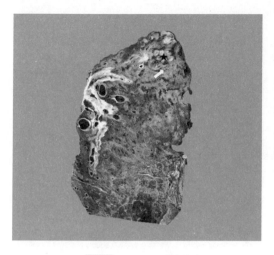

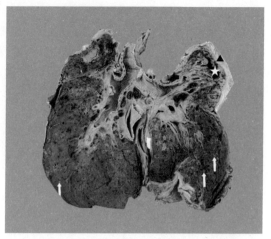

图 14-11　浸润型肺结核病
Fig. 14-11　Infiltrative pulmonary tuberculosis

图 14-12　浸润型肺结核病伴急性空洞
Fig. 14-12　Infiltrative pulmonary tuberculosis with acute cavitation

（4）慢性纤维空洞型肺结核（图14-13）：肺上叶大部分被破坏，形成巨大的空洞（★），空洞壁为较厚的组织形成，内壁粗糙，附有灰黄色的干酪样坏死物质；其余肺组织被大量纤维组织替代，下叶有多数支气管播散的病灶（➡）；胸膜纤维组织增生，胸膜明显增厚；肺组织整体质地变硬，又称为硬化性肺结核。

Chronic fibrous cavitary pulmonary tuberculosis（Fig. 14-13）：Most of the upper lobes of the lungs are destroyed to form huge holes（★）, the hollow walls are formed by thicker tissues, the walls are rough, with gray-yellow caseous necrotic substances; the rest of the lungs are replaced by a large number of fibrous tissues, and the lower lobes are mostly bronchial disseminated lesions（➡）; pleural fibrous group tissue hyperplasia, pleura significantly thickened; the overall texture of lung tissue hardened, also known as sclerosing pulmonary tuberculosis.

（5）肺结核球（图14-14）：肺切面上可见直径等于或大于2 cm的球形病灶（★）。病灶境界清楚，病灶中心为干酪样坏死，周围有纤维组织包绕（➡）。

Pulmonary tuberculoma（Fig. 14-14）：There is a round lesion with a diameter more than 2 cm on the cut surface（★）. The lesion has a clear boarder and undergoes caseation in the center. The periphery of lesion is wrapped by connective tissue（➡）.

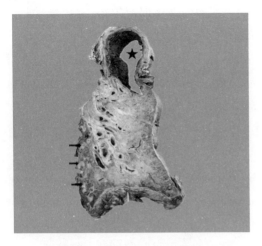

图 14-13　慢性纤维空洞型肺结核

Fig. 14-13　Chronic fibrous cavitary pulmonary
tuberculosis

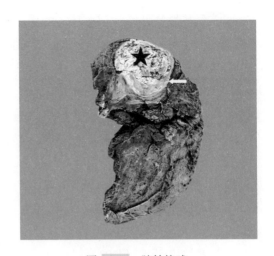

图 14-14　肺结核球

Fig. 14-14　Pulmonary tuberculoma

（三）肺外器官结核病 Extrapulmonary tuberculosis

（1）肠结核病（图 14-15）：回肠黏膜面有数个溃疡（图 14-15a），呈椭圆形或带状，其长轴与肠的长轴相垂直（➡）。从背面观察，有的标本有肠狭窄（➡）（图 14-15b）。

Tuberculosis of the small intestine（Fig. 14-15）：There are several ulcers on the mucous membrane of ileum（Fig. 14-15a），which are oval or strap-shaped with their long axes perpendicular to the long axis of lumen（➡）. Some ileums have narrowed lumens（➡）from the back（Fig. 14-15b）.

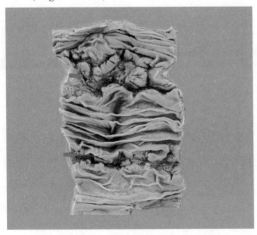

a. 溃疡型 Ulcerous type

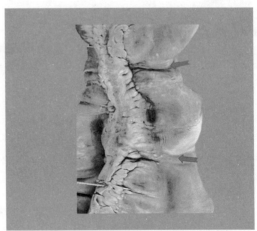

b. 肠腔狭窄 Intestinal stenosis

图 14-15　肠结核病

Fig. 14-15　Tuberculosis of the small intestine

（2）结核性脑膜炎（图14-16）：大脑底部蛛网膜下腔内液体混浊不清，有灰黄色炎性渗出物积聚。有的标本在大脑侧沟附近可见散在的针尖大结核病灶（➡）。

Tuberculous meningitis（Fig. 14-16）：It is turbid in subarachnoid space on the base of brain, enriched with grey-white inflammatory exudate. Points of tuberculous lesions can be found around the lateral cerebral sulcus（➡）.

（3）小脑结核球（图14-17）：小脑半球内有一个直径约1.5 cm的球形病灶（★），切面为灰黄色干酪样坏死。

Cerebellar tuberculosis（Fig. 14-17）：There is a spherical lesion（★）about 1.5 cm in diameter in the cerebellar hemisphere, with grey to yellow-colored caseous necrosis on the cut surface.

（4）肾结核病（图14-04）：肾体积变大，外形不整。切面可见肾实质被大量破坏，有干酪样坏死及空洞形成。肾盂、肾盏也被破坏变形。

Tuberculosis of the kidney（Fig. 14-04）：The enlarged kidney has an irregular surface. On the cut surface, renal parenchyma is destroyed, which are replaced by caseous necrosis and cavities. Renal pelvis and calices are also distorted.

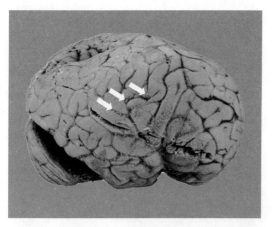
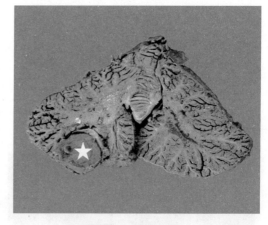

图 14-16　结核性脑膜炎　　　　　　　　图 14-17　小脑结核球
Fig. 14-16　Tuberculous meningitis　　　Fig. 14-17　Cerebellar tuberculosis

（5）肠系膜淋巴结结核（图14-18）：标本是肠与肠系膜粘连的切面。肠系膜淋巴结由于结核病变而高度肿大，并有大片干酪样坏死，淋巴结互相粘连融合成团块状（➡），与肠管粘连而难以分离。

Tuberculosis of the mesenteric lymph nodes（Fig. 14-18）：It is the cut surface from the intestine and adhered mesenterium. Note that the mesenteric lymph nodes are enlarged obviously due to tuberculosis, with massive caseous necrosis, which result in the fusion of adjacent lymph nodes（➡）and adherence with intestines.

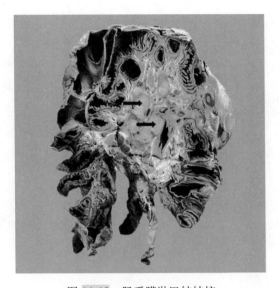

图 14-18　肠系膜淋巴结结核

Fig. 14-18　Tuberculosis of the mesenteric lymph nodes

（三）伤寒病 Typhoid fever

（1）伤寒肠（髓样肿胀期）（图 14-19）：回肠黏膜面有肿胀隆起的、椭圆形的集合淋巴结，以及呈圆形的孤立淋巴结（★）。

Intestinal typhoid fever（medullary swelling stage）（Fig. 14-19）：There are raised oral Peyer's patch and round solitary lymph nodules on the mucous membrane of ileum（★）.

（2）伤寒肠（坏死期）（图 14-20）：肿胀隆起的淋巴组织内发生坏死，坏死物呈淡灰黄色，多以中心部开始逐渐扩大至整个淋巴组织（★）。

Intestinal typhoid fever（necrotic stage）（Fig. 14-20）：The swelling lymphatic tissue undergoes necrosis, which is white-grey colored and expands from the center to the complete tissue（★）.

（3）伤寒肠（溃疡期）（图 14-21）：回肠中有一椭圆形溃疡，边缘整齐，底部光滑，可见暴露的环肌层，溃疡的长轴与肠的长轴相平行（➡）。

Intestinal typhoid fever（ulcerous stage）（Fig. 14-21）：There is an oval ulcer in the lumen of ileum, which has an orderly margin and glossy bottom（➡）. The circular muscle layer is exposed. The long axis of ulcer lays in parallel with the long axis of intestine.

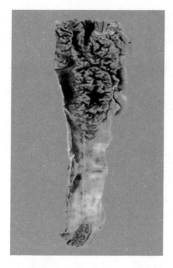
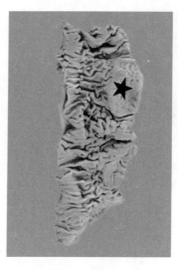
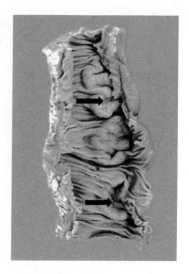

图 14-19　伤寒肠（髓样肿胀期）　　　　图 14-20　伤寒肠（坏死期）　　　　图 14-21　伤寒肠（溃疡期）

Fig. 14-19　Intestinal typhoid　　　Fig. 14-20　Intestinal typhoid　　　Fig. 14-21　Intestinal typhoid
　　fever（medullary swelling stage）　　　fever（necrotic stage）　　　　fever（ulcerous stage）

（四）细菌性痢疾 Bacillary dysentery

急性细菌性痢疾（图 14-22）：结肠黏膜面附着一层粗糙、污秽的灰褐色或灰黄色假膜（★），有的在脱落后形成浅表小溃疡（➡）。固定较好的新鲜标本可见溃疡间黏膜充血、水肿及炎症变化。

Acute bacillary dysentery（Fig. 14-22）：A layer of rough white-grey pseudomembrane is attached to the mucous membrane of colon（★）. Small superficial ulcer forms after the separation of membrane（➡）. Hyperemia，swelling and inflammatory change can be found in fresh and well-prepared specimens.

（五）寄生虫病 Parasitic disease

（1）阿米巴痢疾（图 14-23）：结肠黏膜面有多个散在分布的小米粒大的溃疡开口（➡）。有的溃疡融合，开口大；有的溃疡口边缘附着灰黄色坏死物。溃疡之间的组织一般仍属正常。

Amebic dysentery（Fig. 14-23）：There are many spots of ulcers disseminated on the mucosa of colon（➡）. Some of these ulcers fused to a bigger one，and the opening is large. Some has yellow necrotic substance attached to them. The tissue between ulcers appears normal.

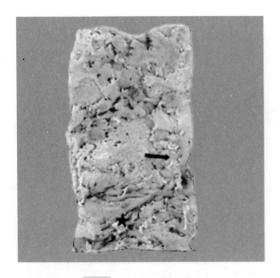

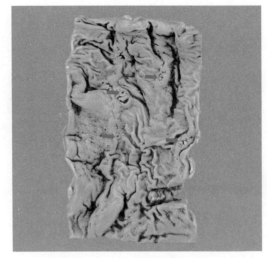

图 14-22 急性细菌性痢疾
Fig. 14-22 Acute bacillary dysentery

图 14-23 阿米巴痢疾（肠阿米巴病）
Fig. 14-23 Amebic dysentery（Amebiasis of the intestine）

（2）阿米巴肝脓肿（图 14-24）：肝切面上，各脓肿大小不一（直径 1 ~ 6 cm，数目 1 ~ 3 个不等），脓肿周围组织受压迫，有的脓肿已穿破肝包膜。本标本上可见一个直径 6 cm 左右的脓肿（★），脓肿壁粗糙，腔内充满灰黄色的坏死物（➡）。

思考题：脓肿穿破肝包膜后有什么危险？

Hepatic amebic abscesses（Fig. 14-24）：On the liver cut surface, there are several amebic abscesses with varying size（1 – 6 cm in diameter, and 1 – 3 in number）, and the surrounding liver tissue is repressed by the abscess. Some abscesses even perforate the Glisson's capsule. In this case, an abscess about 6 cm in diameter is found（★）and the abscess has rough walls, and filled with white-grey necrosis（➡）.

Question：What is the risk if the abscess perforates the Glisson's capsule?

（3）慢性血吸虫病肠（图 14-25）：结肠黏膜粗糙，有浅表小溃疡。部分黏膜增生，呈小息肉样（➡）。黏膜下层纤维性增厚，浆膜面附脂肪组织。

Chronic schistosomiasis of the colon（Fig. 14-25）：There are many superficial ulcers on the coarse mucosa of the colon. Part of the mucosa undergoes hyperplasia, which gives a polypoid appearance（➡）. There is fibrous thickening in the submucosa and adipose tissue in the serosa is hyperplastic.

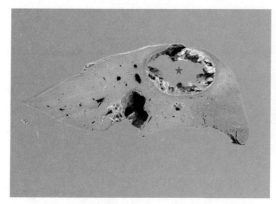

图 14-24　阿米巴肝脓肿

Fig. 14-24　Hepatic amebic abscesses

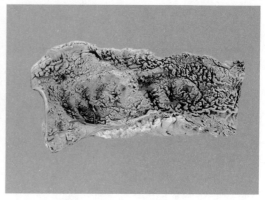

图 14-25　慢性血吸虫病肠

Fig. 14-25　Chronic schistosomiasis of the colon

（4）肠血吸虫性肉芽肿伴癌变（图 14-26）：标本中部或下部为血吸虫性肉芽肿改变（➡）。近肛门部组织呈灰白色，高低不平，并浸润破坏肌层，此即为癌变区域（★）。

Intestinal schistosomiasis granuloma with malignant transformation（Fig. 14-26）：There is a schistosomiasis granuloma change in the middle or lower part of intestine（➡）. Note that some of these tissue near the anus exhibits a white-grey, uneven, which infiltrates to the muscularis and gives evidence for malignant transformation（★）.

（5）血吸虫性肝硬化（图 14-27）：肝脏体积缩小，表面高低不平，有散在沟纹（➡），形如地图样。切面门脉区结缔组织增生，呈树状分布（▲），故有"干线性肝硬化"之称。

Schistosomiasis cirrhosis（Fig. 14-27）：The liver has a reduced size, and the surface is uneven, with scattered grooves（➡）. On the cut surface, hyperplastic connective tissue is found lining around the portal triad（▲）, namely the "pipe stem cirrhosis".

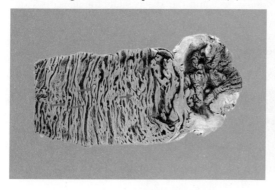

图 14-26　肠血吸虫肉芽肿伴癌变

Fig. 14-26　Intestinal schistosomiasis granuloma
with malignant transformation

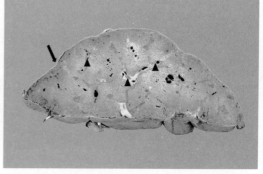

图 14-27　血吸虫性肝硬化

Fig. 14-27　Schistosomiasis cirrhosis

三、组织切片观察 Observation of tissue slides

（一）结核病 Tuberculosis

（1）粟粒性肺结核（图14-28）：肺组织中可见散在、境界清楚的结节状病灶——肉芽肿（＋）。多数结节中央为红染、无结构、细颗粒状的干酪样坏死（➡），周围为增生的上皮样细胞（类上皮细胞）（▲），并杂有少数朗罕氏巨细胞（★），外层有淋巴细胞（◀）及少量纤维组织包绕。

Miliary pulmonary tuberculosis（Fig. 14-28）：There are many well-defined nodules scattered in the pulmonary parenchyma, which is the "granulomas" of tuberculosis（＋）. Granulomas are composed of caseous necrosis in the center, which has an amorphous granular pink appearance（➡）；the transformed macrophages of epithelioid cells（▲）and Langhans giant cells（★）, along with lymphocytes（◀）and a small amount of fibroblast in the periphery.

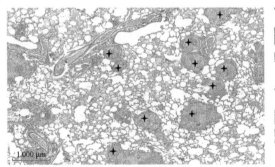

低倍视野 low magnification　　　　高倍视野 high magnification

图 14-28　粟粒性肺结核
Fig. 14-28　Miliary pulmonary tuberculosis

（2）干酪性肺炎（图14-29）：肺组织呈大片干酪样坏死伴有单核细胞浸润（★）。原有的肺组织结构不清，周围肺泡腔内有大量浆液性纤维素性渗出物（➡）及大量单核细胞与淋巴细胞。

Caseous pneumonia（Fig. 14-29）：There is a massive area of caseous necrosis along with monocyte infiltration in the lung tissue（★）. The original structure of lung tissue is disrupted, with serous or fibrinous exudate（➡）, and numerous monocytes and lymphocytes infiltrating in the alveolar space.

（3）肾结核（图14-30）：肾组织中可见散在的结核结节（★）及慢性炎症细胞。

Renal tuberculosis（Fig. 14-30）：Scattered tubercles（★）and chronic inflammatory cells are found in the kidney.

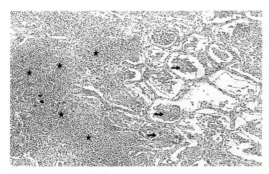

图 14-29　干酪性肺炎
Fig. 14-29　Caseous pneumonia

图 14-30　肾结核
Fig. 14-30　Renal tuberculosis

（4）淋巴结结核（图 14-31）：局部淋巴结正常结构（▲）消失，被大量红染、无结构的颗粒状物（★）取代，表明组织坏死彻底，不残留原来的组织结构。

Tuberculosis of the lymph nodes（Fig. 14-31）：Normal structure（▲）of lymph nodes disappeared，which is replaced by massive amorphous pink granules（★），indicating the complete necrosis of tissue and dispearanced of normal architectures.

（二）细菌性痢疾 Bacillary dysentery

急性细菌性痢疾（图 14-32）：结肠黏膜表面覆盖一层假膜（★）。假膜由纤维素及其网罗的坏死组织与炎症细胞碎屑组成，并可见大量黏液（▲）。黏膜及黏膜下层充血、水肿，并伴有炎症细胞浸润（➡）。部分假膜脱落后形成浅表不规则溃疡。

Acute bacillary dysentery（Fig. 14-32）：There is a layer of pseudomembrane on the superficial surface of colonic mucosa（★）. The pseudomembrane is composed of cellulose，which traps derris from necrotic tissue，inflammatory cells and a large amount of mucus（▲）. There is hyperemia and edema，along with inflammatory infiltration in the mucosa and submucosa（➡）. Superficial irregular ulcers are formed after part of the pseudomembrane fall off.

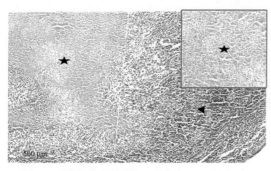

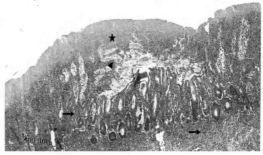

图 14-31　淋巴结结核
Fig. 14-31　Tuberculosis of the lymph nodes

图 14-32　急性细菌性痢疾
Fig. 14-32　Acute bacillary dysentery

（三）伤寒 Typhoid fever

（1）肠伤寒（图 14-33）：回肠黏膜固有层的淋巴组织增生（★），其中有大量增生的单核细胞。有的细胞吞噬了红细胞、淋巴细胞或细胞碎片，此种细胞常被称为"伤寒细胞"。伤寒细胞聚集，形成伤寒小结。肠系膜淋巴结内可见类似病变。

Intestinal typhoid fever（Fig. 14-33）：There is lymphoid hyperplasia in the lamina propria of ileum mucosa（★）, which is composed of a large amount of monocyte. Some of these cells phagocytosed debris from erythrocyte, lymphocyte or other cells, and transformed into the "typhoid cells". The typhoid nodule is formed by the enrichment of typhoid cells, which could also be seen in mesenteric lymph nodes.

（2）伤寒淋巴结病变（图 14-34）：淋巴结肿大，淋巴窦内可见大量增生的单核细胞及"伤寒细胞"（➡）。

Typhoid lymph node lesion（Fig. 14-34）：Lymph nodes are enlarged, and a large number of proliferating monocytes and "typhoid cells"（➡）are seen in the lymphatic sinus.

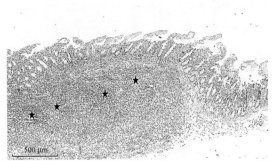

图 14-33 肠伤寒
Fig. 14-33 Intestinal typhoid fever

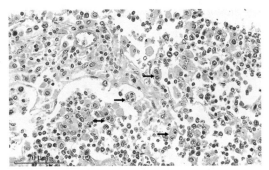

图 14-34 伤寒淋巴结病变
Fig. 14-34 Typhoid lymph node lesion

（四）性传播性疾病 Sexually transmitted diseases

尖锐湿疣（图 14-35）：表皮角质层轻度增厚，几乎全为角化不全细胞（▲），棘层肥厚，有乳头状瘤样增生（★）。表皮浅层可见凹空细胞（➡）；凹空细胞较正常细胞大，胞浆空泡状，核增大居中，染色深，可见双核或多核。真皮层可见炎症细胞浸润。

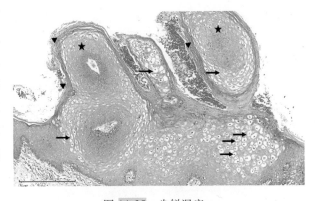

图 14-35 尖锐湿疣
Fig. 14-35 Condyloma acuminata

Condyloma acuminata（Fig. 14-35）：The epidermis stratum corneum is slightly thickened, and occupied by parakeratotic cells（▲）. Acanthosis and papillomatous hyperplasia undergoes in the epithelium（★）. The typical koilocyte（➡）is larger than normal cells, which is characterized by cytoplasmic vacuolization and double or multiple nuclei in the center with dark staining. Inflammatory cells' infiltration is found in the dermis.

（五）寄生虫病 Parasitic disease

（1）阿米巴痢疾（图14-36）：结肠黏膜可见坏死灶（▲），并呈潜掘至黏膜下层。有的坏死灶中的红染、无结构的坏死物已大部分被排至肠腔，形成口小底大的烧杯状溃疡（★）。坏死灶或溃疡周围可见到较多的阿米巴滋养体（➡）及一些淋巴细胞、单核细胞浸润，各层血管充血；有的静脉中已有阿米巴滋养体侵入（◀）。

Amebic dysentery（Fig. 14-36）：Necrotic lesions（▲）are found in the colonic mucosa, which sneaked into the submucosal layer. When the necrotic tissue is discharged to the lumen, it forms a flask-shaped ulcer with a narrow neck and board bottom（★）. Many amebic trophozoites（➡）can be found in the necrotic lesions and ulcers, which even invades into the veins（◀）. Lymphocyte and monocyte infiltration is found in the necrotic lesions, and hyperemia is present in different layers.

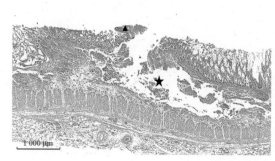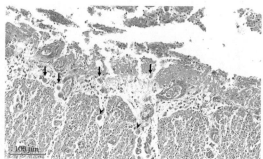

图 14-36　阿米巴痢疾

Fig. 14-36　Amebic dysentery

（2）血吸虫病肠（图14-37）：结肠黏膜固有层及黏膜下层有较多血吸虫卵沉着，并可见虫卵结节：①嗜酸性脓肿：中央为红染的坏死组织及虫卵（➡），周围有大量嗜酸粒细胞围绕（★）。②假结核结节：中央为变性坏死或钙化的虫卵，周围有异物巨细胞，有的正在吞噬或已吞噬了血吸虫卵，外围有上皮样细胞、纤维组织包绕及炎症细胞浸润。③纤维化结节：数枚钙化虫卵（◀）伴有大量纤维组织增生（▲）。

Schistosomiasis of the colon（Fig. 14-37）：Schistosome eggs are found in the lamina propria and submucosa of colon. The composition of "egg nodule" is as the following：① Eosinophilic abscess：Necrotic tissue and eggs（➡）are found in the center, which is surrounded by eosinophils（★）．② Pseudotubercle：Degenerated or necrotic eggs are found in the center，with foreign-body giant cells in the surrounding，which is responsible for the phagocytosis of eggs．Epithelioid cells，fibrous tissue and inflammatory cells are present in the periphery．③ Fibrous nodule：calcified eggs（➚）are wrapped with massive fibrous tissue（▲）．

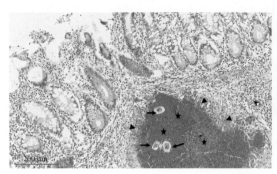
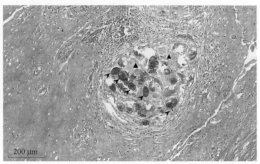

图 14-37　血吸虫病肠

Fig. 14-37　Schistosomiasis of the colon

（3）血吸虫病肝（图 14-38）：汇管区可见嗜酸性脓肿。请自己学习判断各种结构。

假结核结节：中央为变性坏死或钙化的虫卵（➡），周围有异物巨细胞（★），有的正在吞噬或已吞噬了血吸虫卵，外围有上皮样细胞（➚）、纤维组织包绕及炎症细胞浸润。

Schistosomiasis of the liver（Fig. 14-38）：Eosinophilic abscess is present in the portal area．Please try to recognize them．

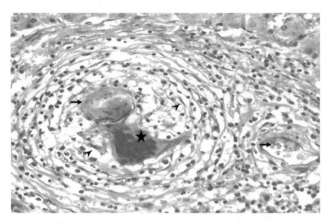

图 14-38　血吸虫病肝

Fig. 14-38　Schistosomiasis of the liver

Pseudotubercle：Necrotic eggs are found in the center（➡），which are surrounded by foreign-body giant cells（★）．Epithelioid cells（➚），fibrous tissue and inflammatory cells are present in the periphery．

四、　病例讨论 Case discussion

患者，男，23 岁，因"右足踇趾化脓数天，畏寒、发热 2 天"入院。入院前数天右足踇趾跌伤后感染化脓，自行切开引流。

体格检查:体温39.5℃,脉搏130次/分,呼吸40次/分,血压80/50 mmHg。急性病容,神志模糊,双肺可闻及较多湿啰音。全身皮肤有多数瘀斑,右小腿下部发红、肿胀,有压痛。

实验室检查:白细胞计数 25.0×10^9/L,中性粒细胞0.75。

入院后即使用激素、抗生素治疗。入院后12 h出现低血压休克,于第三日死亡。

尸检:全身散在皮下瘀斑,踇趾外侧有一约1.5 cm长的外伤创口,表面有脓性渗出物覆盖。双肺重量增加,有多数大小不等的出血区及灰黄色粟粒大的脓肿。双肺上叶有硬结性病灶,右上叶硬结内有一直径约0.8 cm的大空洞。镜下见空洞壁由类上皮细胞、朗汉斯巨细胞、淋巴细胞及成纤维细胞构成,近腔面有干酪样坏死,抗酸染色检查见少许结核杆菌。

A 23-year-old male patient was admitted to the hospital for suppuration of the thumb of his right foot, and chills and fever for two days. The patient had injury and suppuration on his feet, and operated on his thumb by himself.

Physical examination: Temperature 39.5 ℃, pulse 130 times per minute, breath 40 times per minute, blood pressure 80/50 mmHg. The patient was weak and ambiguity, and moist crackles were found on both lungs. Ecchymosis was found all over the body. The right lower limb was red and swollen.

Laboratory examination: White blood cell count 25.0×10^9/L, Neutrophils 0.75. The patient was treated with glucocorticoid and antibiotics immediately, but had hypotensive shock 12 hours later and died three days after admission.

Autopsy was performed. There was extensive ecchymosis was found all over the body, and a 1.5 cm-long wound covered with purulent exudate was found. There was increased weight of both lungs, and lesions of hemorrhage and spots of yellow abscesses were found. There were hard nodules on the upper lobes of both lungs, and a 0.8 cm big cavity on the upper lobe of right lung. Microscopily, the wall of cavity consisted of epithelioid cells, Langham's giant cells, lymphocyte and fibroblast. Approach to the surface of cavity, there was caseous necrosis and some tubercle bacillus was found.

问题 Questions

（1）死者生前患有哪些疾病（病变）？

What diseases did the patient have before death?

（2）请解释这些疾病（病变）是如何发生、发展的。

Please explain the pathogenesis and development of these diseases.

五、 思考题 Questions

（1）试述结核病的基本病变、转归和发病机制。

Please illustrate the basic pathologic changes, prognosis and pathogenesis of tuberculosis.

（2）试述成人型肺结核的各型特点及转归。

Please explain the characteristics and results of different types of adult tuberculosis.

（3）伤寒的基本病变及其临床病理联系是什么？

What are the basic pathological changes and clinical features of typhoid fever?

（4）流行性脑脊髓膜炎的基本病变特点与其临床特点的联系是什么？

What are the basic pathological changes and clinical features of epidemic cerebrospinal meningitis?

（5）乙型脑炎的病变特点有哪些？

What are the pathological changes of encephalitis B?

（6）名词解释：原发综合征、干酪样肺炎、结核球、冷脓肿、关节鼠、伤寒细胞、中毒型菌痢、噬神经细胞现象、Waterhous-Friedricsen 综合征。

Please explain: primary complex, caseous pneumonia, tuberculoma, cold abscess, joint mouse, typhoid cell, toxemic bacillary dysentery, neuronophagia and Waterhous-Friedricsen's syndrome.

（7）按下表鉴别原发性与继发性肺结核病。

Please find the differences between primary and secondary tuberculosis according to the table below.

	原发性肺结核 Primary tuberculosis	继发性肺结核 Secondary tuberculosis
发病年龄 Age		
病灶起始部分 Original lesion		
肺门淋巴结 Hilar lymph node		
病理变化 Pathological change		
主要散播方式 Way of dissemination		

编写 Written by：万珊 Wan Shan　谢芳 Xie Fang

中文审核 Chinese proofreader：邓敏 Deng Min

英文审核 English proofreader：刘瑶 Liu Yao

附录 部分章节大体标本二维码

第一章 细胞和组织适应与损伤

阿米巴肝脓肿　　　　　肺结核　　　　　　干性坏疽

肝细胞水肿　　　　肝脂肪变性　　　淋巴结结核病-干酪样坏死

脑积水　　　脾脏包膜玻璃样变　　脾脏凝固性坏死

前列腺增生症　　　肾凝固性坏死　　　肾萎缩-肾盂积水

心脏萎缩

第二章　损伤的修复

创伤性神经纤维瘤

骨折愈合-畸形愈合

皮肤疤痕-一期愈合

第三章　局部血液循环障碍

肠出血性梗死

动脉瘤伴血栓形成

二尖瓣狭窄伴附壁血栓

肺出血性梗死

股动脉内血栓

夹层动脉瘤

流行性出血热

慢性肺淤血

慢性肺淤血-肺褐色硬变

慢性肝淤血-槟榔肝

门静脉血栓

脾脏贫血性梗死

肾贫血性梗死

心脏贫血性梗死

第四章 炎症

慢性扁桃体炎

肺炎性假瘤

急性重症肝炎

阑尾及各种阑尾炎

慢性胆囊炎伴结石

皮肤瘘管

皮肤痈

气管白喉

纤维素性心包炎-绒毛心

第五章 肿瘤

肠壁脂肪瘤

大肠溃疡性癌

多发性平滑肌瘤

肝海绵状血管瘤

肝细胞性肝癌

肝转移性绒毛膜癌

膈肌种植性转移癌

脚趾恶性黑色素瘤

卵巢囊腺瘤

卵巢黏液性囊腺瘤

囊性成熟性畸胎瘤

皮肤乳头状瘤

脾转移性癌

乳腺浸润性癌

软骨肉瘤

肾盂尿路上皮乳头状癌

纤维瘤

小肠平滑肌肉瘤

眼底肿瘤-视网膜母细胞瘤

阴茎恶性黑色素瘤

阴茎鳞状细胞癌

第六章　心血管系统疾病

动脉粥样硬化性固缩肾

二尖瓣关闭不全

二尖瓣关闭不全伴狭窄

二尖瓣狭窄

二尖瓣狭窄伴
附壁血栓

二尖瓣狭窄伴三
尖瓣关闭不全

高血压颗粒
固缩肾

高血压性心脏病伴
主动脉粥样硬化

夹层动脉瘤

脑出血（1）

脑出血（2）

心脏萎缩

亚急性感染性心内膜
炎-主动脉瓣赘生物

正常心脏

正常心脏-
右心室

正常心脏-主动脉左心室

正常心脏-左心部分

正常左心室-二尖瓣

主动脉粥样硬化

第七章　呼吸系统疾病

大叶性肺炎

肺疤痕癌

肺气肿（1）

肺气肿(2)

肺源性心脏病

硅肺(1)

硅肺(2)

硅肺(3)

硅肺-3 期伴结核

小叶性肺炎(1)

小叶性肺炎(2)

支气管扩张

周围型肺癌(1)

周围型肺癌(2)

第八章　消化系统疾病

肠癌(1)

肠癌(2)

肠癌-隆起型

肠癌-外生型

大结节性肝硬化(1)

大结节性肝硬化(2)

大结节性肝硬化伴肝癌

胆汁性肝硬化

肝细胞癌

肝硬化伴肝癌

急性重症肝炎（1）

急性重症肝炎（2）

浸润型胃癌

巨块型肝癌

溃疡型胃癌

慢性肥厚性胃炎

慢性萎缩性胃炎（1）

慢性萎缩性胃炎（2）

慢性胃溃疡伴急性出血

慢性胃溃疡病

弥漫浸润性胃癌

十二指肠溃疡穿孔

食管癌

食管癌-溃疡型

食管癌-隆起型

食管癌-髓质型

胃癌

胃癌-浸润型

胃癌-溃疡型（1）

胃癌-溃疡型（2）

胃胶样癌

多发性胃溃疡病

胃溃疡病

胃溃疡慢性穿孔

小结节性肝硬化（1）

小结节性肝硬化（2）

小结节性肝硬化-全肝

小结节性肝硬化伴肝癌

亚急性重症肝炎（1）

亚急性重症肝炎（2）

直肠癌-隆起型

直肠癌-浸润型

直肠癌-溃疡型

第九章　淋巴造血系统疾病

肠恶性淋巴瘤（1）

肠恶性淋巴瘤（2）

肠恶性淋巴瘤（3）

第十章　泌尿系统疾病

膀胱尿路上皮
乳头状癌（1）

膀胱尿路上皮
乳头状癌（2）

急性弥漫性增生性
肾小球肾炎（1）

急性弥漫性增生性
肾小球肾炎（2）

慢性肾小球肾炎-继发
性颗粒固缩肾（1）

慢性肾小球肾炎-继发
性颗粒固缩肾（2）

慢性肾盂肾炎

膜性肾病

肾细胞癌

肾盂尿路上皮乳头状癌

第十一章　生殖系统疾病与乳腺疾病

睾丸精原细胞瘤

卵巢浆液性囊腺瘤

卵巢黏液性囊腺瘤

卵巢黏液性乳头状囊腺瘤

前列腺增生症(1)

前列腺增生症(2)

侵蚀性葡萄胎

乳腺癌

乳腺癌-乳头凹陷

阴茎鳞状细胞癌(1)

阴茎鳞状细胞癌(2)

子宫多发性平滑肌瘤

子宫颈癌

子宫内膜癌

子宫绒毛膜癌(1)

子宫绒毛膜癌(2)

子宫腺肌瘤

子宫黏膜下平滑肌瘤

第十二章　内分泌系统（甲状腺）疾病

甲状腺癌

甲状腺乳头状癌（1）

甲状腺乳头状癌（2）

甲状腺腺瘤

甲状腺肿

结节性甲状腺肿（1）

结节性甲状腺肿（2）

结节性甲状腺肿伴囊性变

第十三章　神经系统疾病

化脓性脑膜炎

脑出血

脑积水

脑转移性肿瘤

神经鞘瘤

小脑胶质瘤

第十四章 感染性疾病

肠阿米巴病

肠结核(1)

肠结核(2)

肠伤寒(1)

肠伤寒(2)

肠伤寒-坏死期

肠粘连伴肠系膜淋巴结结核

肺结核空洞

急性肺粟粒性结核(1)

急性肺粟粒性结核(2)

结核球

浸润性肺结核病

淋巴结结核

慢性肺粟粒性
结核病

慢性纤维空洞型肺结核-
硬化性肺结核病

肾结核病(1)

肾结核病(2)

细菌性痢疾

小脑结核球

血吸虫肠

血吸虫肠伴癌变

血吸虫肝

血吸虫肝伴门静脉血栓

原发性肺结核病

参 考 文 献

［1］步宏,李一雷. 病理学［M］. 9 版. 北京:人民卫生出版社,2018.

［2］罗塞. Rosai & Ackerman 外科病理学［M］. 10 版. 郑杰,主译. 北京:北京大学医学出版社,2014.

［3］翟启辉,周庚寅. 病理学［M］. 北京:北京大学医学出版社,2015.

［4］KUMAR V, ABBAS A K, ASTER J C. Robbins basic pathology ［M］. 10th ed. Philadelphia:Elsevier, 2017.

［5］KUMAR V, ABBAS A K, ASTER J C. Robbins and Cotran pathologic basis of disease ［M］. 9th ed. Philadelphia:Elsevier Saunders,2015.